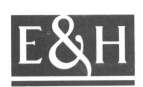

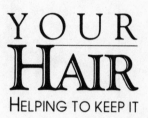

YOUR
HAIR
HELPING TO KEEP IT

YOUR HAIR

HELPING TO KEEP IT

*Treatment and
Prevention of
Hair Loss for
Men and Women*

NEIL S. SADICK, M.D.
DONALD CHARLES
RICHARDSON
and the Editors of Consumer Reports Books

CONSUMER REPORTS BOOKS
A DIVISION OF CONSUMERS UNION
Yonkers, New York

Copyright © 1991 by Neil S. Sadick, M.D., Donald Charles Richardson, and the Editors of Consumer Reports Books

Published by Consumers Union of United States, Inc., Yonkers, New York 10703.

Library of Congress Cataloging-in-Publication Data
Sadick, Neil S.
  Your hair : helping to keep it : treatment and prevention of hair loss for men and women / Neil S. Sadick, Donald C. Richardson and the editors of Consumer Reports Books.
    p.   cm.
  Includes bibliographical references and index.
  ISBN 0-89043-450-6
  1. Baldness—Prevention.   2. Hair—Care and hygiene.
I. Richardson, Donald Charles.   II. Consumer Reports Books.
III. Title
RL 155.S33   1992   92-12200
616.5'46—dc20   CIP

Design by Ruth Kolbert

First printing, May 1992

Manufactured in the United States of America

Figure 2-1, Male Pattern Baldness, Copyright © 1991, adapted from *Consumer Reports*, September 1988

Your Hair: Helping to Keep It is a Consumer Reports Book published by Consumers Union, the nonprofit organization that publishes *Consumer Reports*, the monthly magazine of test reports, product Ratings, and buying guidance. Established in 1936, Consumers Union is chartered under the Not-for-Profit Corporation Law of the State of New York.

The purposes of Consumers Union, as stated in its charter, are to provide consumers with information and counsel on consumer goods and services, to give information on all matters relating to the expenditure of the family income, and to initiate and to cooperate with individual and group efforts seeking to create and maintain decent living standards.

Consumers Union derives its income solely from the sale of *Consumer Reports* and other publications. In addition, expenses of occasional public service efforts may be met, in part, by nonrestrictive, noncommercial contributions, grants, and fees. Consumers Union accepts no advertising or product samples and is not beholden in any way to any commercial interest. Its Ratings and reports are solely for the use of the readers of its publications. Neither the Ratings, nor the reports, nor any Consumers Union publication, including this book, may be used in advertising or for any commercial purpose. Consumers Union will take all steps open to it to prevent such uses of its material, its name, or the name of *Consumer Reports*.

The ideas, procedures, and suggestions contained in this
book are not intended to replace the services of a
physician. All matters regarding your health require
medical supervision. You should consult with your
physician before adopting any of the procedures in this
book. Any applications of the treatments set forth in this
book are at the reader's discretion, and neither the
author nor the publisher assumes any responsibility or
liability therefor.

C O N T E N T S

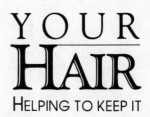

YOUR
HAIR
HELPING TO KEEP IT

Introduction

Throughout history, people have been obsessed with hair, equating luxurious locks with youth, virility, strength, beauty, and sensuality. For as long as records have been kept, hair has been described as a sexual object. Indeed, hair condition, styling, and length have been among the more charismatic standards of beauty in virtually every civilization. Hair has also played an important part in the religious and cultural rituals of many societies.

Baldness, by contrast, has been viewed as a negative personal attribute. This is more than simply the flip side of the emphasis on a beautiful full head of hair; societies have long shaved the heads of prisoners, traitors, or other lawbreakers as a mark of shame or punishment. Romans cut the hair of adulteresses and traitors, and the French Resistance cut the hair of women who collaborated with the occupying German army during World War II. Hair has also been removed specifically to downplay sexual attractiveness. The shaved bald spot on the tops of monks' heads, creating the style known as tonsure, was adopted by early Christians in an effort to make the monks less sexually attractive.

Although ancient attitudes toward hair may seem bizarre today, there are still rituals and practices associated with the cutting, arranging, and coloring of hair. The way a person's hair is worn can be an indication of social position, even a political statement. For example, during the 1960s and 1970s male students often chose to wear their hair long to express their antiestablishment sentiments. Unusual hairstyles and hair colors among the young have often been declarations of independence and freedom from conformity.

Even for the individual not intending to make a statement with his or her hair, the condition, appearance, and, particularly, presence of hair maintain a distinct mystique that is every bit as fascinating and influential today as it was thousands of years ago. If there is any doubt that contemporary society places a high value on hair, simply leafing through newspaper or magazine articles and advertisements will show just how important hair is to the general population. Along with complex and apparently endless collections of hair-grooming preparations, there are often advertisements for hair-growth products, procedures, and recent findings that are, for the most part, a triumph of hope over experience and reality. But this doesn't matter. To make hair look good, especially to keep it or grow it again, many men and women will do absurd and even occasionally dangerous things. It would seem that, along with the fountain of youth, the search for a baldness remedy is among humankind's great quests.

Prehistoric humans had a general covering of hair over their bodies that conserved heat and provided camouflage from predatory animals. Over time human beings have largely lost the body hair that still protects the skins of other primates. And, regardless of the fact that in modern society no one really *needs* hair for health, the absence of a full head of hair is at best frustrating, at worst psychologically damaging. Whether caused by a physical condition, medical procedure, or inherent physiological change, hair loss can be traumatic and stressful for both men and women. Research has shown that people who lose their hair often suffer from low self-esteem and lack of self-confidence.

Baldness *is* viewed negatively by the general public. Research has shown that balding men are sometimes judged to be five years older than their actual age and thought to be less assertive in business and personal relationships, less successful, even less likable.

The emotional impact of hair loss, combined with the loss itself, can actually create the conditions by which more hair is lost. Although worrying about hair loss does not in itself precipitate the loss, stressful situations such as operations, injury, acute illness, or severe emotional situations (such as the death of someone close) may exacerbate tendencies to lose hair in predisposed individuals. Both men and women who experience extreme stress about their scalp problems can suffer from diffuse shedding of hair beginning three to four months after a stressful episode. Stress may also play a role in precipitating *alopecia areata,* a disease of the hair follicles in which people lose well-defined patches of hair. This condition can show up as the loss of small patches of hair or, in its most severe manifestation, as total baldness all over the body.

It is interesting that, despite our obsession with hair, many primary-care physicians do not examine hair as part of a regular physical. And this oversight can be a mistake. Hair, and its condition, can indicate vitamin and protein deficiencies, thyroid conditions, anemia, collagen vascular diseases such as lupus, infections and infestations, even AIDS. And, although the greatest percentage of men who lose their hair are victims of hereditary baldness *(andro-genetic-dependent alopecia),* a number of factors— including stress, systemic medical conditions, traumatic injury, or psychiatric conditions such as eating disorders (anorexia nervosa) and plucking of one's own hair *(trichotillomania)*—can contribute to hair loss in both men and women. Many of these conditions are treatable.

Your Hair: Helping to Keep It investigates the full range of causes of hair loss. It examines the means by which people try to regain their hair (some realistic, some ridiculous), details the methods that may come into use to replace lost hair, and discusses the many products available for hair grooming.

PART ONE

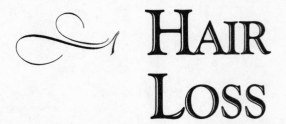 HAIR LOSS

1

How Hair Grows

Science fiction often portrays futuristic people, both male and female, as totally bald. This creative device is based on the observation that the evolution of the human animal is marked by a progressive loss of hair. Drawings of early humankind indicate that at one time most of the human body was covered with hair. This hair provided warmth and insulation against the elements. It could also, through color and pattern, create a camouflage from predators and enemies. Over time, as the survival needs of the species changed, human beings, unlike other animals, lost much of this covering of hair. Of course, evolution is never a perfect engineer, and there are many individuals, fully evolved as we can be sure, who still have extensive body hair (see chapter 6).

A striking feature of contemporary human hair is that, despite its sparse distribution relative to that found in other primates, it is by no means vestigial (rudimentary or nonfunctional) and is indeed both plentiful (humans have more hair follicles per unit of skin area than most higher primates) and capable of growing to great length.

Hair follicles can first be recognized at nine weeks of development and show up most prominently on the eyebrows, upper lip, and chin. Hair follicles develop in a head-to-toe *(cephalocaudal)* direction, until the entire fetus is covered with soft, fine, poorly pigmented hair. This prenatal hair is called *lanugo* hair. It is replaced soon after birth by *vellus* hair, a fine, minimally pigmented hair that has limited growth potential. Vellus hair contains the inner hair core and most often appears on the face, scalp, and forearms. It continues to grow throughout life, often covers much of the body, and is usually not visible to the naked eye. The thick, fully pigmented hair most people recognize as "real" hair is called *terminal* hair.

✎

HAIR NUTRITION

Because hair growth requires a rich supply of oxygen and nutrients provided by blood vessels around the base of the hair follicle, it is vital that the necessary environment for healthy hair growth be provided. The major component of terminal hair is protein (65 to 95 percent by weight), and the predominant amino acids are sulfur-containing cystine, cysteine, arginine, and citrulline. The cross-linkage of these amino acids gives hair its rigid quality. Other components include water, fats (lipids), pigment, and trace elements.

∽

VISIBLE HAIR

The part of the hair we see and recognize as hair is actually the *hair shaft*. This shaft is composed of three concentric layers: an outer casing called the *cuticle;* a sheath inside the cuticle called the *cortex;* and an innermost *medulla,* the basic structural core.

The hair grows out of a *follicle,* a pouchlike structure below the skin containing a compound sheath. A single follicle is capable of producing lanugo, vellus, and terminal hairs. The active growing zone of hair is the hair *bulb,* a protrusion in the sac at the bottom of the hair follicle. Within this sac is the *papilla,* containing the hair *matrix,* a compartment actively reproducing all components of the hair shaft.

The shape of the hair is usually related to the race of the individual. For example, the straight hair of most Asians is round in cross section. The cross section of Caucasian hair is usually oval. The curly hair of people with African ancestry shows a flattened oval in cross section. Both Caucasian and African hair tend to be smaller in diameter than Oriental hair.

Texture

The strength and body of a person's hair are determined by a number of factors. Basically, the strength of individual strands of hair comes from the hair cortex, which is made up of keratin fibers in a sulfur-rich matrix. The stiffness and resilience are determined by the amount and binding interaction of the sulfur-containing amino acids. The body in a head of hair is determined by four interrelated components: the density, stiffness and resilience, diameter, and physical interactions of the individual hair fibers.

Body

The density of hair fibers on the scalp simply refers to the number of follicles per surface area. On average a newborn has 1,135 hair follicles per square centimeter of scalp area. Between 3 and 12 months, this number is reduced to about 795 per square centimeter. And between the ages of 20 and 30, there are usually about 615 hair follicles per square centimeter.

The diameter of each hair fiber is important in this context. Scalp hair diameter varies from .02 to .04 millimeters. And, although it is clear that the number of hair follicles diminishes, there is a rapid increase in the diameter of hair with age, particularly through the first three to four years of life. It is interesting to note that curly hair has more body than straight hair. This is because of two factors. First, individual curly hairs tend to be thicker than straight hairs. And, second, curled hair fibers cannot help but bounce against one another, piling higher on the head.

Physical interactions among the hair fibers also contribute to body. This is the one controllable aspect of hair body, determined as it is by the care a person takes with grooming hair, or, for that matter, the damage that can be brought about by poor care.

Human beings are born with all their hair follicles in place. The amount of hair a person has on his or her head and body is therefore established at birth. Some of these follicles are programmed to change in size over time, but no new hair follicles develop after birth.

There are normally about 100,000 hairs on the human scalp. All hair follicles have identical structures and go through cycles of active growth and rest, although at different times.

∽

HAIR CYCLES

The hair follicle is the only organ in the body that functions as a cyclic growth, no-growth system. The process consists of three phases: anagen, catagen, and telogen.

Anagen Phase

The *anagen* phase is the growing and active part of a hair's life; at any moment 85 to 90 percent of all the hair on the scalp is in this phase. During this phase, reproductive cells grow and expand into the upper part of the hair bulb to form the hair shaft. Single anagen hairs are normally growing; they are not shed. In general, a hair in this phase remains in the scalp an average of 1,000 days. However, it is possible for hairs to stay in the anagen phase for two to six years simply because the hair-growth cycle varies from person to person. During the anagen phase, the

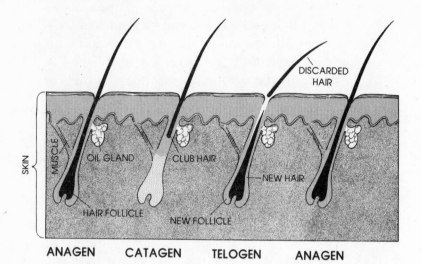

FIGURE **1-1.** *Human Hair. After the active growth period (usually about six years), the follicle disintegrates (up to the surface). The cells in the tip of the root (dermal papilla cells) send a chemical message to the immature cells in the hair bulb, causing them to divide into a new follicle.*

hair shaft diameter increases and the hair reaches its maximum length.

Catagen Phase

During the *catagen* phase, the hair stops growing and begins its transition into the "resting" or telogen stage. In a normal head of hair, 3 to 4 percent of hair is in this phase at any given time. Single hairs are still actively growing and are not shed from the scalp. The catagen phase usually lasts only one to two weeks, during which the hair follicle decreases in volume and pigment formation stops. Also, the lower segment of the hair follicle is destroyed, and the structure of the active, growing part of the hair bulb and matrix cells disappears, creating a *club hair*, a rudimentary structure that forms in the hair shaft as it goes into the resting phase of the cycle.

Telogen Phase

The *telogen*, or resting stage, is the final phase of the hair cycle. Thirteen percent of normal scalp hairs will be in this phase, which lasts five to six weeks. In the telogen phase, the rudimentary regressed inactive hair *(epithelial column)* is further reduced. This hair is short and tends to be shed spontaneously. For the average person, it is normal to lose up to 100 hairs per day. This process is known as *physiological shedding* and is a normal part of a replenishing organ system.

The length of the hair when it reaches the telogen phase varies from person to person and is proportional to the duration of the anagen phase and individual growth rates. At the end of the telogen phase, the hair is shed. New activity in the hair follicle indicates a return to the anagen phase, leading to a new shaft ascending the follicle. The hair that forms behind the regressing telogen hair actually forces the old hair to fall out.

AGE-RELATED CHANGES IN HAIR

Although hair growth, loss, and regrowth is a straightforward biological process, there are some interesting aspects to the cycle. For example, it has been noted that immediately after birth a child loses hair over the front and sides of the scalp in a pattern remarkably similar to adult male pattern baldness. In infancy, to make up for this hair loss, all the hairs lost are replaced by follicles entering the anagen stage.

At birth, a Caucasian child's hair shaft is round, but during the first two years of life it assumes an oval cross section, and this remains through life. Regardless of sex, the cross-sectional area quickly grows to 0.25 millimeters at age 3, but thereafter increases more gradually to 0.40 millimeters at age 17. However, overall hair density is slightly greater in males than in females (199 versus 185 per centimeter). Because females enter puberty earlier than males, they develop and complete an adult pattern of hair sooner.

From the formation of hair follicles in the fetal stage until the person's death, hair pattern is always in a state of transition. The first conspicuous change in normal hair pattern occurs during puberty. The growth of terminal hair on the face, trunk, and limbs is under the influence of androgenetic hormones, their receptors, and enzymes that are involved in the metabolic conversion of hormones.

In the adult, hair maintains a stable pattern for most. However, if there is a genetic predisposition for male pattern baldness, there may be periods of intermittent shedding and changes in hair pattern.

In old age, hair may turn gray, and progressive hair pattern changes may accelerate in genetically predisposed people. The hair shafts at this time may be dry and somewhat brittle, similar to changes in the rest of the skin.

∽
HAIR COLOR

Hair color is controlled by the presence of *melanin*. Depending on its degree of expression, this substance may produce colors varying from gray to yellow-brown to red to black. There are two types of melanin, *eumelanin*, which gives hair black-brown color, and *pheomelanin*, which gives hair auburn or blond color. Also, hair color usually varies according to its anatomical location. For instance, scalp hair is generally lighter than genital hair, and eyelashes are often the darkest hair on an individual.

Hair color is linked to genetic factors. Within the European community, blond and red hair are more common in northern Europeans, whereas black hair appears most frequently among southern and eastern Europeans. Of course, there are wide variations within these basic divisions.

Although the hair of Asians and Africans is predominantly brown-black, hair color among Caucasians varies widely, from the lightest blond through shades of red and brown to black. In addition, hair color among Caucasians changes over time. In a German study of 2,000 6-year-olds and children between 6 and 12, the hair color in the first group was predominantly light (63 percent), while 25 percent had medium-dark hair and 12 percent had dark hair. In the older group, 20 percent had dark hair, 30 percent had medium, and 50 percent had light hair.

The action of the melanin that produces pigment in the skin lessens as an individual ages. Gray hair is usually related to the progressive reduction in function of *melanocyte cells*, those that produce melanin, the active pigment component. Gray hair can be caused by a variety of other conditions as well, including autoimmune disease characterized by underactivity of the adrenal glands (Addison's disease), a loss of hair with a possible autoimmune origin (alopecia areata), and underactive thyroid function (hypothyroidism). Over time the body may produce antibodies against melanocytes, contributing to the graying process. All these disorders may be associated with autoimmune factors, suggesting that there may be an immunologic basis to the graying of hair, although genetic predisposition is usually the most influential factor.

Although gray hairs are usually noticed earlier in those with dark hair, complete graying often takes place earlier in fair-haired people. Gray hair first appears between the ages of 35 and 40 in those of European ancestry, and, by the age of 50, 50 percent of this population's hair is gray. The onset of gray hair is approximately a decade later among those of African descent. A man's hair grays first in his beard and mustache. On the scalp, men's and women's hair grays at the temples first, followed by the crown and, last, the back of the head.

Many instances of premature graying are genetically caused. There are also reports of "sudden graying." Although no scientific proof has survived, folklore suggests that when Sir Thomas More and Marie Antoinette were told they were to be executed, the hair of each turned gray overnight. And it is possible that acute traumas, such as major illness, drug reaction, or severe accident, can lead to rapid graying.

2

Common Causes of Hair Loss

There are many causes of hair loss in both men and women. Some are temporary conditions that may cure themselves. Others may be very complicated, associated with disease or other systemic disorders. Of course, finding the fundamental cause of the hair loss is necessary before any treatment program can be prescribed.

∽

MALE PATTERN BALDNESS (ANDROGENETIC Alopecia)

The most common cause of hair loss for men is male pattern baldness *(androgenetic alopecia)*. This condition, which affects over 30 million men in the United States alone, has been recognized as a disorder since the time of Hippocrates and has received more attention, publicity, and medical investigation than any other kind of hair loss.

The replacement of some adult hairs by fine babylike hairs from puberty onward is an almost universal phenomena, with some degree of normal hair loss occurring in up to 96 percent of adult men and 79 percent of adult women. The hair loss in women, however, is not as significant as in men.

Ninety-five percent of male pattern baldness is linked to heredity. There is a 50 percent chance of children inheriting the trait, with a more likely inheritance when the trait is on the female side of the family.

Male pattern baldness occurs most frequently during puberty, the second decade of life, and the fourth decade. Frequently, the first sign is hair that has fallen out, whether episodically or persistently. The second sign is a noticeable thinning of scalp hair.

The Pattern

The typical pattern of hair loss begins at the frontal hairline. Hair then thins at the crown. Eventually the receding hairline meets the bare crown for the characteristic horseshoe configuration: a central expanse of baldness with a fringe of hair along the sides of the scalp.

This kind of hair loss is gradual. Every hair lost is not lost forever. As the hair passes through its three on-off stages, the follicles become smaller, finer, and shorter. More follicles remain in the resting stage, and there is a gradual conversion of long, thick, pig-

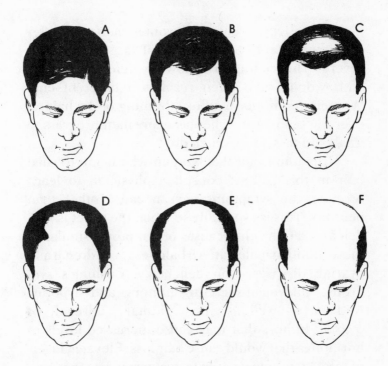

FIGURE **2-1.** *Male Pattern Baldness. Shown in its typical progression, male pattern baldness is by far the most common form of hair loss, eventually affecting two out of three men. Such baldness is inherited—from either the father's or mother's side of the family. It is not caused by poor circulation in the scalp or deficiencies of vitamins.*

mented (terminal) hair to short, fine, lightly pigmented (velluslike) hair, which is much like that on a newborn infant. Although male pattern baldness is usually most noticeable on the head, some people find that other hairy areas of the body, such as eyebrows and the pubic area, are also affected. Usually hair on extremities shows only a decreased rate of growth rather than complete loss.

A smaller percentage of women than men suffer from hereditary baldness, and it is generally less severe. The condition follows a different pattern with women and often reaches a different end. Women first notice a diffuse thinning of the hair all over the scalp. And, whereas many men progress to total baldness, few women do.

It is important that women who begin to shed hair in this pattern consult a physician to learn whether the symptoms have a cause other than heredity. This is especially so when the onset is sudden and rapid. Other causes of symptoms similar to those found in male pattern baldness are adrenal and ovarian diseases, iron deficiency, Cushing's syndrome, androgen-secreting tumors, and hypothyroidism, as well as other pituitary, adrenal, or ovarian tumors that may cause increased levels of hormones that would cause hair loss. Elevated levels of total testosterone, free testosterone, or other hormones can be present. Or decreased hormone levels (sex hormone–binding globulin, luteinizing hormone, follicle-stimulating hormone, and estradiol) may be part of the cause.

Myths and Truths

It is important to face and dismiss the false perceptions that have grown up around hereditary baldness. In neither men nor women is it related to insufficient blood supply, emotional problems, clogging of hair follicles, or poor diet, resulting in vitamin deficiency or increased levels of toxins. Male pattern baldness is directly connected to a combination of genetic and hormonal factors. Those who have this condition have been genetically programmed to develop it. It is exacerbated by male hormones and increased sensitivity of hormonal receptors to normal amounts of androgen, the male hormone believed to be responsible. In patients with the condition there is greater activity of a certain enzyme, 5 alpha reductase, which converts testosterone to its active metabolite (dihydrotestosterone). So men with this kind of baldness have greater enzyme activity and greater capacity to bind hormones at the receptors in the hair follicle. A deficiency of a newly discovered enzyme, armatase, may also play a role.

However, regardless of the often dramatic reduction in follicle size that occurs in male pattern baldness, the follicle itself is not altered in structure, nor does the number of follicles change. The count of hair follicles can diminish for other reasons—for instance, most of us lose follicles as we age. Of course, when we lose follicles and those that remain lose their ability to produce terminal hair, the hair loss is both greater and more noticeable.

To determine the amount of hair a person has lost, doctors use a grading system, the *Hamilton scale* (as modified by Norwood) for men, and a similar system created by Ludwig for women. Although neither of these systems is absolutely precise, both offer a range of classifications for hair loss. In the Hamilton/Norwood system, hair loss is graded from Type I, with mild bifrontal thinning, to Type VII, in which diffuse thinning of the scalp from front to back is noted. In the Ludwig classification, the gradation

moves from mild, which is associated with slight diffuse thinning, to severe, in which there is significant
loss of hair on both the front and back areas of the
scalp. These methods of grading help diagnose
excessive hair loss in individual patients and confirm
that there is some change in the patterns of hair
growth over time in all adults of both sexes.

Although some men experience great stress and
embarrassment over hair loss, they rarely consult a
doctor about the situation. More commonly they ask
help from their hairstylists or try unproven products.
Hippocrates observed around 400 B.C. that "eunuchs
never go bald" (they don't have any testosterone),
but this doesn't mean, as some bald men would like
to think, that they have more testosterone than men
with full heads of hair. While a stylist can help to disguise thinning hair cosmetically—by curling, coloring, and combing—there are a number of medically
proven treatments—including hormonal therapy,
topical and biological drugs, and transplants—available from doctors to treat baldness (see chapters 9
and 10). As previously noted, women who have
hereditary baldness should investigate the possibility
of medical disorder at the first symptoms.

TEMPORARY HAIR LOSS

Along with permanent hair loss resulting from
androgenetic conditions, some common temporary
hair loss conditions can affect both men and women.
While the symptoms—hair thinning and shedding—

may be similar to those experienced in male pattern baldness, other causes of hair loss do not result in the characteristic horseshoe pattern.

For reasons not yet fully understood, evolution and natural selection have determined that human hair grows only to a certain length over several years and is then shed. This is the three-phase cycle described in chapter 1. This metamorphosis of a growing hair into a reduced hair stub is a normal part of the hair life cycle. Although the timing mechanism remains somewhat a mystery, the process is coordinated by a biological clock built into every hair. However, some external factors can actually override the biological clock and thrust a hair follicle into the reduced or resting phase. If large numbers of resting hair follicles are affected at the same time, the condition is called *telogen effluvium*. Telogen effluvium is always triggered by another condition, and it is almost always temporary.

The causes of telogen effluvium fall into two categories. The first is related to bodily functions. For example, pregnancy often causes numerous hair follicles to remain longer than normal in the active growing state, most likely because of the influence of pregnancy hormones. After childbirth, the hormonal restraint is reduced and many hair follicles enter the reduced or resting phase over several weeks. (It has not yet been determined whether the stress of childbirth contributes to telogen effluvium.)

Telogen effluvium is also nearly always present in a newborn baby. During the first six months of life, a child sheds scalp hair. This can happen rapidly, which results in the baby's appearing bald, or it may occur very slowly and be almost imperceptible.

Regardless of the schedule or even the appearance of hair loss, an enormous number of active, growing hairs enter the resting state within months, throwing the hair into a final synchronized molt that establishes the permanent hair.

The first stage of male pattern baldness may be associated with telogen hair shedding. Long, fully grown hairs are shed within the regular hair cycle and usually replaced. At the beginning it is possible to shed many hairs without the loss becoming apparent (a person will usually lose as much as 50 percent of the hair in an area before noticing any loss). If a normal hair is replaced by a normal hair, the hair loss can be attributed to telogen effluvium. However, if the hair follicle produces a miniature hair, it usually marks the onset of male pattern baldness.

Telogen effluvium is not physiological and involves injury or stress to the hair follicles. These traumas can include fever, severe infection, chronic illness, psychological stress, surgery, hypothyroidism and other endocrine disorders, crash or liquid protein diets, and drugs, such as ingested (not topical) vitamin A derivatives, antiepidermal thickening agents, blood thinners (particularly heparin), antithyroid drugs, anticonvulsants, and hormones. Heavy metals such as lead and arsenic also may cause telogen effluvium. Essentially, this category is made up of factors that "insult" the hair follicles.

Although hairs that have entered the resting phase cannot be brought back to the active, growing state, once the physical condition that brings about telogen effluvium is removed, the hair should be able to recycle and regrow within 6 to 12 months.

∽

IMMUNOLOGIC HAIR LOSS
(Alopecia Areata)

Inflammatory diseases that cause an individual's immune system to become overactive can also result in hair loss. Up to 25 percent of the patients experiencing this condition undergo some form of acute psychic trauma before the hair loss. Some people believe that a psychological insult may impair regulation of immune activity and hair follicle growth, although it must be emphasized that this is a hypothesis that lacks scientific substantiation.

In immunologic hair loss, the overactive immune system decreases the number of peripheral blood cells (lymphocyte suppressor/cytotoxic cells), which help regulate and control immunologic activity. This reduction in cells may be the factor that causes the hair to fall out. More recently it has been hypothesized that immunologic hair loss may be related to a defect in regulation of the hair matrix.

Immunologic hair loss is a common disease and affects about 0.5 percent of new patients in dermatologists' offices (approximately 0.05 to 0.10 percent of the general population). It is estimated that 1 percent of the population will, by the age of 50, have experienced immunologic hair loss at some time. There seems to be a genetic component. A family history of the problem is present in about 20 percent of patients. There are reports of identical twins developing the condition simultaneously, and occasionally three or four generations have affected members. The condition affects all races and occurs worldwide.

This condition usually begins as one or more, well-circumscribed areas of hair loss; loss of hair from beard, eyebrows, or the pubic area occurs in 10 percent of patients and may precede scalp involvement. The round or oval patch of baldness (lesion) generally shows skin that is smooth, soft, ivory white, and totally devoid of hair. Along the margins of the centrifugally spreading patch are often tapered hairs that are easily plucked. There is no evidence of scarring on the surface of the skin, which helps to differentiate this disorder from other causes of hair loss. Immunologic hair loss can be present in other patterns, such as a band of rimmed hair loss along the scalp margin *(ophiasis)*, loss of all scalp hair *(alopecia totalis)*, and loss of all body and scalp hair *(alopecia universalis)*. In these cases the prognosis is poor. Long-standing hair loss and associated nail changes also suggest a poor prognosis.

Immunologic hair loss can also be associated with stippling or grooving of the nails as well as changes in the pigment of the remaining hair. Moreover, when the hair regrows it is often initially white, and then regains its normal color.

Although this condition is medically benign, the rapid onset, recurrent episodes, and unpredictable course of immunologic hair loss may profoundly disrupt the lives of those affected. The condition can be acute and short-lived or chronic, with regrowth in some areas and progressive loss in others. It may stabilize with patches that remain unchanged for years, or progress from patchy to total baldness within days or weeks. In one-third of the cases, the initial attack lasts less than six months and in 50 percent less than one year. A resolution of the condition takes place within five years in 70 to 80 percent of patients. However, 20 to 30 percent fail to recover from the initial attack. The factors dictating the unpredictable course of this disorder are unknown, but stress and intercurrent medical illnesses are often noted by physicians who see and treat it.

Although prediction is difficult, it can generally be said that if hair loss is severe and diffuse, the condition appears with associated conditions such as allergy (asthma or hay fever), and it occurs before puberty, the prognosis is poor. Similarly, if there is a rapid progression of hair loss, loss of eyebrows and eyelashes, and severe changes in the appearance of the fingernails, chances of regrowth are small. In its simpler forms, in which hair loss is confined to the one or a few regions, the prognosis is more positive.

The cause of immunologic hair loss is still unknown, although the condition can be associated with autoimmune disorders—such as thyroid disease, vitiligo, and pernicious anemia (anemia associated with vitamin B deficiency), or with hypertension and multiple allergies. It can also be connected to Down's syndrome.

There are several unresolved questions concerning immunologic hair loss. For example, the medical community has not yet established whether this condition—from a mild, patchy form to the wider-spread alopecia totalis and alopecia universalis—is really only one disease. And, although alopecia areata is suspected of being the consequence of an autoimmune problem (the body's immune system interacting against itself), at present there is no direct evidence linking it with other autoimmune disorders. Infection and stress have also been mentioned as possible factors in triggering alopecia areata, although their roles remain controversial.

Often immunologic hair loss takes a benign course and remits spontaneously, without any treatment. There is always the possibility for complete hair regrowth, even for those with extensive (including 100 percent) scalp hair loss for many years. But at present there is no definitive cure for any stage of the disorder, although there are a variety of medical therapeutic methods available for treatment.

Treatment

It must be understood that, while one treatment or another may stimulate hair growth in the affected area, it won't prevent the appearance of the condition on other parts of the head.

CORTICOSTEROIDS These drugs are sometimes tried, either topically (applied on the surface of the affected area) or by injection into the hairless area. In children, corticosteroids are most often applied topically. Oral steroids are used in more severe cases. In many cases, although corticosteroids will cause hair to regrow, when they are stopped the hair will once again fall out. Although topical applications can be administered at home by the patient or a family member, injections of corticosteroids into the scalp, which need to be repeated monthly until full hair growth resumes, must be given by a physician.

TOPICAL IRRITANTS Certain topical irritants and allergens have been used to treat immunologic hair loss. Topical irritants, such as anthralin (a coal tar distillate) and croton oil (an irritant), induce inflammation of the scalp skin, which in turn stimulates hair regrowth. Topical allergens, such as DNCB (dinitrochlorobenzene), induce an allergic contact dermatitis (an autoimmune reaction where the body's immune system becomes activated) on the scalp. Visible hair regrowth occurs in patients 8 to 12 weeks after the application of an irritant substance, and for about 50 percent of patients cosmetically acceptable hair growth follows.

A drawback is that after early success a person may acquire a tolerance to a medication, rendering it ineffective. The practical problems with such treatment include the look of inflammation that irritants often induce and the toxicity of these substances, particularly for patients under 16 years old. Moreover, these treatments are still considered experimental, are not widely available, and have possibly dangerous side effects. These include allergic reactions as well as the more important consideration that DNCB has been shown to have some cancer-potentiating activity in laboratory animals. Patients are advised to avoid topical irritants and allergens unless the condition is otherwise unmanageable.

PUVA Psoralen plus ultraviolet light, known as PUVA, is a combination of medication and exposure to ultraviolet light that can stimulate hair growth. The disadvantages of this treatment are the frequency of treatment required (about three per week) and its toxicity, which includes the possibility of skin cancer caused by photodamage to the skin and cataracts occurring after years of treatment.

MINOXIDIL   Biological response modifiers such as minoxidil in 1 to 5 percent concentrations have achieved positive results in up to 65 percent of patients. It is thought that minoxidil may specifically exert its effect on T lymphocytes and thus be an immune modulatory agent. Another theory is that it may act at the cellular level to stimulate growth and/ or improve cell differentiation in the hair matrix.

It has been noted that increased concentrations produce increased regrowth, but minoxidil treatment requires prolonged therapy. Success may be enhanced by the combination of minoxidil with tretinoin (Retin-A). Systemic absorption of minoxidil is minimal, and there have been no reported significant changes in blood pressure, EKG, or laboratory tests on patients using the medication in concentrations under 5 percent.

The choice of treatment for immunologic hair loss is determined by the age of the patient and the extent of the condition. In about one-third of patients, particularly those with local patches of hair loss, spontaneous regrowth may occur with no medical treatment.

∽

TRAUMATIC HAIR LOSS
(TRACTION Alopecia)

Traumatic, or mechanical, hair loss *(traction alopecia)* is characterized by the presence of short broken hairs, inflammation of the hair follicles *(fol-*

liculitis), and scarring in circumscribed patches at the periphery of the scalp. This condition is actually self-induced and is usually categorized by its causes. For example, brush roller hair loss is caused by a too frequent application of brush rollers, which results in irregular patches of hair loss surrounded by zones of inflammation with broken hairs. Hot comb hair loss occurs most often in women using hot combs to straighten hair, a process that can result in progressive scarring hair loss. Massage hair loss results from overenthusiastic applications of medication to the scalp with firm massage. Brush hair loss can come from overzealous brushing of the hair. Cultural hair loss is the result of particular hair arrangements, such as the tradition among Sikh men of twisting their uncut hair tightly on top of their heads. There have even been cases of cultural hair loss resulting from the tight clips nurses use to hold their caps in place.

The obvious treatment for this kind of hair loss is avoidance of the precipitating factor.

Pulling Out One's Own Hair (Trichotillomania)

In *trichotillomania*, an individual, usually under stress, pulls out his or her own hair. This condition, most common in females between the ages of 11 and 17, has its root in psychological conditions. Studies of people pulling out their own hair have shown that the condition is usually easily eradicated in children, except among those who are mentally handicapped. In adults the treatment can be more difficult and may require extensive psychiatric care.

Stress-Induced Hair Loss

Severe periods of stress may cause hair to be shed, particularly by persons who are genetically predisposed. However, stress as a cause of hair loss has been vastly overstated. Stress has not been shown to be a cause of irreversible baldness. However, other conditions bringing about more permanent hair loss, including immunologic hair loss, male pattern baldness, and the act of pulling out one's own hair, may be exacerbated by stress.

BURNING SCALP SYNDROME

Burning scalp syndrome, a condition in which patients often complain of a feeling of pins and needles, often accompanies androgenetic alopecia and occasionally alopecia areata. The cause of this unusual sensory aberration is not well understood, but doctors divide the condition into cases that cause pain and those that cause itching. Painful scalp can be caused by folliculitis, systemic lupus erythematosus, and bacterial infections. Pruritic (itchy) scalp disorders include psoriasis, seborrheic dermatitis, and fungal infections.

3

Uncommon Causes of Hair Loss

In addition to what may be considered common causes of hair loss, a number of unusual conditions can result in temporary or even permanent hair loss.

∽

BACTERIAL INFECTIONS

The disease-causing bacteria *Staphylococcus aureus* can lead to deep-seated abscesses of the hair follicles *(furunculosis)*. The bacteria is treatable with appropriate antibiotics, such as semisynthetic penicillins or erythromycin.

A *carbuncle* is a deep-seated infection of multiple connecting hair follicles. This condition is often found in the elderly and can be associated with diabetes, cardiac failure, or the use of immune-suppressing medications. The symptoms are baggy, draining nodules on the scalp, which may be associated with reversible hair loss. Carbuncles are most commonly treated with corticosteroids.

Secondary or *tertiary syphilis* can result in hair loss. In secondary syphilis, thinning of the lateral portion of the eyebrow is seen, along with hair loss over the body as well as the scalp. The hair loss is patchy and often diffused throughout the scalp. Appropriate therapy can usually reverse the hair loss. In tertiary syphilis, there may be multiple scarring nodules *(gummas)* on the scalp, with areas of irreversible hair loss. Both secondary and tertiary syphilis are treated with penicillin or other antibiotics.

It is possible for *tuberculosis* to affect the health of the scalp, although this occurs only rarely. There may be reddish brown nodules that leave patches of scarring hair loss in their path. Treatment requires a full investigation to establish whether the disease is present in other organs and then appropriate antituberculosis therapy with sulfone derivatives such as Dapsone, clofazanine, rifampin, or ethionamide.

Leprosy can trigger the loss of body hair, although scalp hair loss is not common with this disease. Such hair loss may be caused by the elevated surface temperature of the skin that results from the disease. Therapy includes internal doses of isoniazid, rifampin, ethambutol, and pyrazinamide.

The bacterial infection *leishmaniasis,* caused by the bite of the sand fly, is most prevalent in the tropics and subtropics and results in lesions forming ulcerative nodules that heal with depressed scars and hair loss. Antimony derivatives are the major therapeutic agents.

The bite of the simulium, a fly that carries a parasite, can cause *onchocerciasis,* a disease characterized by itchy nodules associated with reversible hair loss that develops on the scalp, particularly at the back of the head. This disease is endemic in South and Central America and Africa. If you have visited one of these regions and begin to experience these symptoms, inform your doctor.

VIRAL DISEASES

The most common viral disease causing hair loss is *herpes zoster*. This condition is usually preceded by localized pain and tenderness. It appears first as blisters along a nerve line. There can be temporary hair loss from the affected areas of the scalp. In patients with severe cases, particularly those who also have diseases such as cancer and AIDS, which affect the immune system, this condition may be associated with irreversible hair loss. The hair loss is brought about by scarring of the hair follicles, which destroys the follicles and makes it impossible for them to regenerate. There is often associated pain (postherpetic neuralgia). Antiviral agents such as acyclovir (Zovirax) used to treat herpes zoster have been found to decrease viral shedding and accelerate healing, consequently diminishing hair loss and other adverse side effects of the disease. If herpes is suspected, the person should consult a dermatologist as soon as possible.

FUNGAL DISEASES

The most common fungal cause of hair loss is *ringworm*. This has been a problem for centuries and remains a health risk in areas of the world where antifungal medications are not readily available. The classic lesion produced by the most common organism of this type in the United States, *Trichophyton tonsurans*, includes small boggy plaques or irregular scaling patches studded with black dots and variable hair loss. Although this condition is treatable with appropriate antifungal antibiotics (griseofulvin or ketoconazole), ongoing cases can result in significant hair loss, which may become permanent if left untreated. It is encouraging that most treated cases will have total regrowth. Antifungal and antibiotic side effects, such as headaches and liver problems, must be investigated by taking frequent blood counts. This is especially important for patients using such medications over long periods of time.

HAIR SHAFT STRUCTURAL ABNORMALITIES

There are three main types of hair shaft structural abnormalities: fractures, irregularities, and coiling and twisting.

Fractures

The first type of hair fracture, *trichorrhexis nodosa*, involves a beaded swelling along the hair shaft. This condition is a result of excessive hair brushing, back combing, and other stress-inducing hairstyling methods; application of heat; prolonged ultraviolet exposure; and heavy permanent waving, which inflict mechanical trauma to the hair follicle. The result can be breakage of the hair shaft, resulting in hair loss in areas subjected to the damaging influences. The only treatment is to minimize the outside traumas. In extreme cases the cure can take as long as two to four years.

Another variety of hair fracture, *trichoschisis*, also caused by mechanical trauma, shows up as a clean transverse fracture across the hair shaft, through the cuticle and cortex. This fracture is often noted in congenitally brittle hair, which has a low sulfur content. Treatment, as one would expect, includes avoiding mechanical trauma to the hair.

A condition in which the hair is bent over but does not break all the way across *(trichoclasis)* does not suggest any underlying disease and is usually helped by more gentle treatment of the hair.

"Bamboo hair" *(trichorrhexis invaginata)* is a nodular expansion of the hair shaft in which a knob-like deformity is noted. This is a unique structural condition resulting from either trauma or one of several congenital syndromes most commonly associated with a congenital scaling disorder *(ichthyosis)*.

Normally known as split ends or the "frizzies," *trichoptilosis* is characterized by a longitudinal splitting or fraying of the hair ends. This condition most often occurs in hair damaged by excessive styling. Gentle hair care is the best treatment.

Irregularities

One frequently observed irregularity of the hair shaft shows up as longitudinal ridging and grooving. This condition may be a normal variant or may occur as part of certain congenital syndromes.

In the familial "uncombable hair syndrome,"

the hair shafts are triangular in cross section. Although biotin has been helpful in some of these cases, the condition is essentially untreatable.

Other irregularities include a condition in which the growing hair divides into two separate shafts *(pili bifurcati)*, another in which two to eight hair matrices and papillae with separate internal root sheaths emerge from one follicular canal *(pili multigemini)*, another that causes ringed hairs showing alternating bright and dark bands in individual hair shafts *(pili annulati)*, and yet another that displays elliptical nodes with intervening tapered constrictions *(monilethrix)*. For these conditions, gentle hair care is desirable. Also, vitamin A derivatives such as etretinate have been helpful in some cases.

Coiling and Twisting

In this condition *(pili torti)*, the hair shaft is flattened and twisted through 180 degrees on its own axis, resulting in a spangled or beaded appearance. The hair shafts are brittle, break off easily, and do not achieve normal length. The condition is often congenital and appears with other defects, such as widely spaced teeth and incompletely developed enamel, nail dystrophy, corneal opacities, horny plugged hair follicles, and ichthyosis.

SCARRING HAIR LOSS

Scarring hair loss *(scarring alopecia)* occurs either in certain areas of the scalp where hair is lost and never grows back or occasionally where a full head of hair is lost and never returns. Various causes lead to the condition.

Hereditary Disorders and Developmental Defects

Scarring hair loss can be caused by an embryological defect noted near the top *(vertex)* of the scalp (*aplasia cutis*) or by localized frontal scalp baldness and skin hardening (Romberg's syndrome). Frontal baldness can also develop early in childhood because of multiple cysts or blisters on these sites. Other medical conditions that may cause scarring hair loss include a disorder characterized by brown, warty plaques (Darier's disease); a genetic disease associated with blisters on hairy and nonhairy skin (epidermolysis bullosa); and a disorder associated with bone disease (Albright's syndrome). These unusual diseases are most commonly diagnosed after consultation with a dermatologist.

Infections

Tuberculosis, syphilis, and pathogenic bacteria may cause scarring baldness, as can fungal infections, viral infections of the herpes group, and protozoal infections such as leishmaniasis.

Tumors

Both benign tumors and malignant skin cancers such as basal cell cancer, squamous cell cancer, lymphomas, and metastatic tumors can cause scarring baldness.

Physical and Chemical Agents

Although radiation (X-ray) in low doses usually does not cause permanent hair loss, high doses of radiation can result in irreversible baldness. Also, caustic agents such as alkalis may damage or destroy hair follicles, leading to scarring hair loss. Burns may be sufficiently severe to destroy hair follicles, and drugs, such as quinacrine and para-amino salicylic acid, have been associated with this condition. Prolonged ultraviolet exposure (sunlight) has not been associated with hair loss.

∽

DRUG-INDUCED HAIR LOSS

Although drug-induced baldness is most often confined to the scalp, other areas, such as the eyebrows, axillary, pubic, and general body regions may also be affected. The only method of determining whether a hair-loss condition is related to a particular drug is to stop the medication. Most often the hair loss will be reversed once the medication is discontinued.

Among the drugs that can adversely affect hair growth are the following:

- Allopurinol, used for the treatment of gout
- Amphetamines

- Androgens
- Anticoagulants. All anticoagulants cause hair loss in a high percentage of patients. One study in which heparin was tested resulted in 50 percent of the study group losing significant hair. Forty-two percent of the group were found to be affected after using sodium warfarin. And a combination of the two resulted in 78 percent of the patients suffering hair loss.
- Drugs used in cancer chemotherapy. This treatment causes hair loss by inhibiting reproduction of the hair follicle. The condition first appears as loss of the active, growing hair but may later change to loss of the rudimentary hair. The extent of hair loss depends on how much of the chemotherapy drug gets to the hair follicle. Applying ice and cold packs around the scalp may somewhat reduce this side effect. Hair loss caused by chemotherapy is temporary.
- Antithyroid medications. Medications that inhibit the synthesis of thyroid hormones are all capable of producing hypothyroidism, a result of which is hair loss.
- Bismuth. Once used to treat syphilis, this drug has been related to hair loss.
- Borates
- Bromocriptine, which regulates prolactin function
- Psychiatric medications, such as Haldol and lithium
- Anticonvulsant medicines, such as trimethadione

- Antihypertensive medications, such as captopril and beta blockers
- Anticholesterol medications, such as clofibrate and nicotinic acid
- Oral contraceptive therapy. Some women notice diffuse loss of hair two to three months after they stop taking birth control pills.
- Antiparkinsonism medications, such as L-Dopa and Ritalin
- Heavy metals, such as gold, mercury, and thallium
- Retinoids, vitamin A derivatives used to treat acne and psoriasis
- Salicylates, as in high-dose aspirin therapy

Anyone suffering from hair loss while taking any of these drugs should be sure to notify the examining physician.

OTHER HAIR and SCALP PROBLEMS

4

Local Diseases of the Hair and Scalp

A variety of diseases and localized conditions can affect the scalp directly by causing inflammation of the hair-bearing skin or by producing growths. These lesions interfere with the normal physiological environment of hair and thus lead to irregular patterns of growth and shedding. Some are minimal and some significant in their pathology. But they have a common underlying result: interference with normal hair patterns and hair growth. These should not be confused with male pattern baldness, which follows a particular configuration.

Three categories form the basis of localized disorders: inflammatory, infectious, and growth or proliferative conditions.

∽

INFLAMMATORY SCALP DISORDERS

Dandruff (Seborrhea)

Although very common, flaking of the scalp is not a normal condition. If the skin of the scalp flakes off, the condition is called *seborrhea* or dandruff. Dandruff affects up to 25 percent of the population. It is caused by abnormal regulation of sebaceous glands and is included in the eczema group of inflammatory conditions of the scalp. Flaking with inflammation of the scalp is called *seborrheic dermatitis*.

Dandruff is characterized by an excessive production of sebum, the semifluid secretion of the sebaceous glands. In this condition, the patient complains of excessively greasy and often unmanageable hair that is not only not helped by shampooing but actually sometimes worsened by it.

However, excess greasiness does not always result in dandruff. Some patients have naturally occurring excess sebum excretion that causes their hair to be unacceptably greasy but may not result in flaking. Men with common baldness may complain of excessive greasiness of the scalp when the greasiness is no greater than average but simply more apparent because of their hair loss.

Simple dandruff, in men and women, often represents increased androgenetic activity that is nothing more than an expression of genetic individuality. But in women the symptoms associated with dandruff should not be left without medical evaluation. Excess greasiness when it accompanies severe acne, hirsutism, and signs of male pattern baldness can indicate the presence of an endocrine abnormality or gynecological tumor.

Currently, there is no cure for dandruff. In some European countries, shampoos containing estrogen are often prescribed and found helpful. However, because these products cause increased activity of glandular structures such as the breasts and uterus, with associated risks of malignancy, they are not considered acceptable in the United States. American physicians treat dandruff with shampoos containing sulfur, salicylic acid, or zinc pyrithione, which act as anti-inflammatory agents, and "keratolytic agents," which minimize scale accumulation and help control the clinical symptoms associated with dandruff.

Scaling Dermatitis (Seborrheic Dermatitis)

This condition is characterized by large, greasy, yellowish scales with crusts, beneath which the scalp is red and moist. In addition, scaly patches can occur behind the ears, in the beard area, on the chest, and on the T zone of the face. Occasionally there may be involvement of the genitalia, which have large numbers of sebaceous glands. This condition also may produce small cysts along the eyelid margins.

The sebum excretion rate is not elevated in this disease, but the sebum has a different composition, with decreased amounts of free fatty acids and higher amounts of triglycerides and cholesterol.

The cause of this scaling condition is unknown, although a genetic predisposition is suspected. It is possible that it is an inflammatory by-product of another condition. Researchers have associated superficial fungi such as *Pityrosporon* yeasts with this type of scaling. The possibility remains the subject of much controversy and scientific investigation.

This dermatitis can be present when AIDS or parkinsonism is diagnosed. Even stress or coronary artery disease can be precipitating factors. There are some indications that this kind of scaling is linked to geographic variations. The condition occurs more often in temperate climates than in tropical ones, although the extent to which climatic and environmental influences play a role is, like the actual cause of the condition, not known.

The condition is treated with shampoos containing sulfur, salicylic acid, zinc pyrithione, and crude coal tar, as well as steroid scalp lotions, antifungal (imidazole) shampoos, and phenol and saline solutions. These agents may decrease inflammation and scaling and associated itching of the scalp. The antifungal agents are employed because superficial fungi are now suspected of playing a role in some cases.

The scalp should be shampooed at least two to three times a week until the inflammation and scaling are under control. In some individuals, daily shampooing may be required. And, because of the chronic and recurring nature of the condition, the patient may find the need to return to the treatment periodically.

Psoriasis

In *psoriasis* the cells of the skin replicate at a too rapid, uncontrolled rate. This genetically determined disease affects 0.5 percent of the population and usually first appears when a person reaches his or her thirties. Psoriasis is characterized by silvery plaques and thickened scales on the scalp. In severe cases, which can result in hair loss, heaped-up scales may extend beyond the hair margin. Although these symptoms may sound similar to those of dandruff, psoriasis is actually quite different. Psoriasis has heaped-up scales, may include involvement beyond the hair margins, and appears in other areas of the body, including the eyebrows, knees, buttocks, umbilicus, and nails.

Although genetics plays a major role in this condition, it is felt to have several causes for its abnormal regulation of cell regrowth and replication. The resulting increased cell reproduction does not increase hair growth. Rather the diameters of the hair shafts are diminished. Psoriasis may also be triggered by stress, infection—especially upper-respiratory infections (particularly in children)—or a distinctive form of arthritis. And drugs such as lithium, withdrawal of corticosteroids, and cardiac medications such as beta blockers may exacerbate the disease.

In the simplest cases, the treatment is the same as for dandruff—a salicylic acid and sulfur-based shampoo is prescribed. If inflammation persists, a steroid scalp lotion or gel can be introduced. In cases where thickened, heaped-up scales prove resistant to these shampoos, coal tar shampoos or solutions, vegetable or peanut oil preparations, and phenol and saline solutions can be used. These act as anti-inflammatory and scale-dissolving agents, as well as decrease the replication of cells. The commonest cause of treatment failure is that individuals do not complete or carry out their treatment properly.

Eczema

Eczema is an inflamation of the scalp associated with scaliness, redness, oozing, and crusting. Eczema itself does not cause hair loss. However, the itching associated with the condition may cause patients to rub or scratch their heads so vigorously that hair loss results. The most common types of eczema—allergic and atopic—appear as an inflammation of the scalp that brings about itching and scratching and thus secondary hair loss. There may be oozing, crusting plaques on the scalp, with associated scaling. Because there is an allergic component to eczema, it usually appears with one or more atopic allergic disorders—asthma, hay fever, running nose—and there is usually a family history of at least one or more allergies. The treatments include steroid lotions, gentle shampoos, antihistamines, and efforts to avoid known or suspected allergens.

Contact Dermatitis

Whereas eczema is a localized manifestation of a systemic problem, symptoms of *contact dermatitis* appear at the exact location where the offending agent touches the skin. There are two forms: irritant dermatitis and allergic contact dermatitis.

Irritant dermatitis is a nonimmunologic condition caused by ongoing applications of a given substance. One common cause is a substance found in permanent wave solutions and bleaching agents.

Allergic contact dermatitis is an immunologic reaction to a particular product. Although some individuals experience an immediate allergy to a substance such as a shampoo, hair dye, rinse, men's hair cream, perfume, lanolin, or preservative, it is also possible to develop an allergy to a variety of products over time. The fibers, adhesives, and laurel oils in hair nets, headbands, and wigs can also cause allergic contact dermatitis.

Contact dermatitis shows up as itchy, crusting, scaling plaques and oozing areas of the scalp. However, severe cases of allergic contact dermatitis may be associated with hives or occasionally anaphylactic shock, a systemwide allergic reaction that can be life threatening.

Since hair dye is one of the most common causes of contact dermatitis of the scalp, it is customary to patch-test (apply a small amount of dye to the skin on the back or arm) to demonstrate the safety of the dye to be used. Treatment includes topical application of steroid lotions and systemic steroids in severe cases.

Hair Casts

Hair casts are marked by accretions of yellowish white specks in the hair and scalp. Although this material is sometimes mistaken for the scales of dandruff or even the nits of head lice, it really represents the residue of certain inner structural fragments of hair that build up on the scalp. There is no known definitive cause for hair casts, but the condition has been linked to scaling disorders of the scalp, such as seborrheic dermatitis and psoriasis. A sex-linked inheritance factor has also been suggested. Traction hairstyles and excessive hair spraying have been studied as possible causes of the condition.

Treatments include lotions containing sulfur or salicylic acid scale-dissolving (keratolytic) preparations. These substances may cause local irritation.

Shampoos that remove scalp scaling are also used. Intensive and prolonged brushing and combing are necessary to slide casts off the affected hair. In treatment, great emphasis is placed on gentle care of the scalp area, because tight hairstyles and overuse of hair spray are felt to play an important role in causing this problem.

∽

INFESTATIONS

Head Lice

Occurring most commonly among children, *head lice* are easily transmitted among people in large close groups, such as schools, although lice may also be caught by direct contact with infected brushes, caps, or combs.

The female head louse is a small, wingless insect, 3 to 4 mm in size, that is parasitic on warm-blooded animals. On human beings, it attaches firmly to the hair shaft, usually on the back of the scalp. Head lice cause itching. Because irritating the area can lead to secondary bacterial infection, the patient needs to avoid scratching. If the infection is left untreated, it may cause malodorous pus.

Head lice are simple to diagnose; eggs, known as *nits*, can easily be seen with a hand lens or Wood's light (an ultraviolet light source). Treatments include topical applications of 1 percent lindane shampoo, 10 percent crotamiton lotion, 5 percent pyrethrin, or 0.5 percent malathion. Physostigmine and fluorescein drugs have been effective as alternative treatments for pediculosis (lice) of the eyebrows. These treatments should be used cautiously because of possible local irritation or neurological dysfunction from extended use.

These agents are usually left on for three to seven minutes and then washed off. This process kills the active live organism. Nits can then be removed from the scalp by drawing a fine-tooth comb through the hair. It is suggested that there be no direct contact with the eggs and that the clothes and bedding used while the patient was infected be thoroughly washed.

∽

PROLIFERATIVE GROWTHS

A variety of growths can appear on the scalp and result in hair loss.

Benign Epidermal Growths

Warty growths on the scalp *(epidermal nevi)* may be associated with localized patches of hair loss. This may occur on a genetic basis and can be associated with other problems, such as seizures and mental retardation. Especially because basal cell cancers may develop secondarily in these lesions, surgical excision is the treatment.

Warty Plaques (Seborrheic Keratoses)

Most often seen in the elderly, warty plaques *(seborrheic keratoses)* may occur in younger people as well. The brown, greasy, warty plaques are often seen first on the face and scalp. When they occur suddenly or become inflamed, they may be a sign of an underlying malignancy. These keratoses are removed by freezing techniques (cryosurgery) or burning of the lesions and then scraping off the remains (electrodesiccation and curettage). Laser therapy is also used.

Senile Keratoses (Actinic Keratoses)

Occurring secondary to sun exposure, these lesions are initially described as senile keratoses (or *actinic keratoses*). They are precancerous and appear as dry, scaling patches with adherent crusts. Ten to 15 percent of these keratoses turn into squamous cell skin cancers. Hair loss does not usually accompany these lesions, although small areas of hair loss may occur as a consequence of chronic picking of the lesions themselves. The treatment includes cryosurgery (freezing with liquid nitrogen), electrosurgery, and fluorouracil (a chemotherapy agent) applied topically. This drug can cause local irritation.

Cutaneous Horns

These horny projections in the scalp arise on top of many lesions, including viral warts, epidermal nevi, seborrheic keratoses, actinic keratoses, and squamous cell cancers. Treatment options include cryosurgery and electrosurgery. A biopsy should always be performed to be sure that there is no underlying cancerous condition. These lesions are rarely associated with hair loss.

Cysts

Enlarged, firm, compressible nodules on the scalp, *cysts* are caused by closure and inflammation of the hair follicles. Cysts may become secondarily infected, and the pressure from these lesions can cause localized areas of hair loss. Treatments include incision and drainage as well as surgical removal.

Malignant Epidermal Growths

Because the scalp is part of the skin, it can be the site of many of the cancers that affect other areas of the skin. Many types of skin cancer are completely curable if treated in a timely fashion, so it is essential that any sore that does not seem to heal—any growth, crusty area, mole, or discolored area of the scalp—be examined by a dermatologist.

Tumors with hair differentiation, sebaceous gland tumors, and sweat gland tumors may appear as enlarging nodules with ulcerations on the scalp and be associated with localized areas of hair loss.

BASAL CELL CANCERS These represent approximately one-third of all cancers and three-quarters of all nonmelanoma skin cancers. They appear as smooth, translucent, slowly enlarging nodules with blood vessels at the surface. When these tumors are suspected, a biopsy should be taken.

BOWEN'S DISEASE   A cancer within the epidermis, Bowen's disease shows up as a thickened plaque on the scalp. It occurs in areas of sun damage and is especially evident in balding men. Bowen's disease may advance into squamous cell cancer. The plaques are most often treated by surgical removal. People with a history of arsenic ingestion from well water or arsenic-containing medicines (at one time utilized in treating asthma or syphilis) are especially susceptible to developing these lesions.

SQUAMOUS CELL CARCINOMAS These hardened ulcers or plaques can appear in sites of burns or X-ray damage. In as many as 5 to 10 percent of the cases, they metastasize to other organs.

Nevi moles can be of particular concern in this respect. A proliferation of melanocyte cells is known as a *nevus*. Most of these lesions develop during childhood or early adult life. Medical treatment is often sought because their appearance has changed over time, or they have enlarged, causing combs to catch in them. Atypical moles with irregular surface, border, and color characteristics are called *dysplastil nevi*. The moles may occur on a familial or sporadic basis and are felt by many researchers to be associated with an increased risk of transformation into malignant melanoma. If they are clinically irregular, they should be removed as a precaution.

MALIGNANT MELANOMA   Melanoma is the most common cause of skin cancer death. As a consequence of greater exposure to sunlight, the incidence of malignant melanoma is increasing. Some people also have a genetic predisposition to them. Thirty to 50 percent of melanomas arise in pigmented moles. In the scalp, where 1 to 3 percent of all melanomas occur, they often arise in congenital melanocytic nevi (see preceding section). Melanoma of the scalp is often associated with spreading of the tumors to distant sites of the body (early metastases) and poor prognosis.

Malignant melanoma appears as a pigmented patch or nodule—brown, black, or red—with irregular surface and border characteristics. The color changes in the mole are often irregular and variegated. Immediate medical evaluation should be sought if a suspicious mole is noticed.

Although the incidence of malignant melanoma continues to increase, the mortality rate remains stable, because so many physicians are more aware of the risks and alert to the first indications of the condition. However, it must be noted that many physicians still do not regularly examine their patients' scalps, so it is prudent to ask your doctor for this checkup. In addition, to minimize the risk of developing malignant melanoma, the patient should reduce sun exposure.

Tumors of the Connective Tissue and Blood Vessels

Growths of the supporting tissue of the skin and blood vessels may produce space-occupying masses leading to subsequent hair loss.

NEUROFIBROMATOSIS (VON RECKLINGHAUSEN'S DISEASE)   This is a disease of the peripheral nerves and associated structures. Inherited as a dominant trait, it occurs in 1 in 2,500 to 3,000 births and appears as "elephant man"–like soft nodules with compressible centers (buttonhole sign). This condition may affect the skin and other organ systems and is associated with café-au-lait spots on the skin in addition to the neurofibrous lesions. Eye involvement and multiple central nervous system tumors may also occur. Neurofibromas may appear as growths with associated hair loss on the scalp. They may be treated by surgical excision or, more commonly, be removed with a carbon dioxide laser.

PROLIFERATIONS OF BLOOD VESSELS (HEMANGIOMA/ VASCULAR NEVI)   These may appear as flat lesions that occur in 20 to 30 percent of newborn babies as a port wine stain on the scalp. Because these marks do not spontaneously disappear, they may be treated with laser therapy.

Another manifestation is a raised lesion or "strawberry mark" (hemangioma), which may continue to enlarge for three to four years after birth. About 50 percent of these lesions disappear spontaneously by age five. Enlarging of this strawberry mark may be associated with localized areas of hair loss. It can be treated with systemic steroids when it is rapidly enlarging and threatening to impinge on a vital structure. The pulsed dye laser and argon laser are the treatments of choice. Cryosurgery and surgical excision are alternatives.

CANCERS METASTATIC TO THE SCALP   The first sign of an otherwise asymptomatic metastatic carcinoma (internal cancer that has spread from the kidney, breast, lung, stomach, colon, ovary, or prostate) may be for the disease to metastasize through the bloodstream or lymph nodes in the scalp. This kind of cancer first appears as one or more nodules that may ulcerate or bleed. If this situation is suspected, a biopsy should be performed immediately.

All vascular lesions on the scalp should be examined by a physician. In addition to diagnosing and treating possible life-threatening conditions, a physician can distinguish among problems that have a similar appearance. Port wine stains, for example, that do not resolve spontaneously can be differentiated from strawberry marks, which may, allowing a patient to make informed choices about treatment.

The treatment of cutaneous vascular disorders has been undergoing revolutionary changes with the advent of a new generation of highly specific laser systems. Utilizing yellow and blue-green laser light and "robot" laser-scanning devices, it is now possible to destroy vascular lesions selectively with minimal or no damage to other cutaneous structures and to lighten port wine stains significantly. Improved clinical techniques using only topical anesthesia, reduce pain, greatly decrease risk of scarring, and allow treatment of patients at any age.

5

Systemic Conditions Affecting the Scalp

Certain diseases that attack other parts of the body can occasionally result in either temporary or permanent hair loss. Anyone trying to determine the cause of his or her hair loss should consider the possibility of a systemic problem and should certainly mention the presence of any such problem to the examining physician. Although in some cases the hair loss cannot be reversed until the underlying condition has been addressed, often the hair loss can be treated directly with good results. Even if the cause is a life-threatening illness, already diagnosed and treated, there is no reason to ignore hair loss. Looking as well as possible can lift one's spirits and ease the burden of coping with other problems.

Reversible hair loss is possible in situations where only the normal cycling of hair growth has been interrupted or where an inflammation interferes with hair growth but doesn't destroy the hair follicles.

Chronic inflammations and scarring scalp diseases can cause deep-seated destruction of the hair follicles and thus make regrowth impossible. Scarring, in particular, destroys the hair follicle structures so they can no longer grow hair. However, some inflammatory diseases are reversible if they are caught early enough and if treatment is begun before the hair follicle is totally destroyed.

✍

METABOLIC DISORDERS

Post-Febrile Hair Loss

People who have suffered high fevers (about 39°C, 102°F or above) can experience severe hair loss 8 to 10 weeks after the first damaging bout of fever. This post-febrile shedding recycles the hair into the resting phase, much like telogen effluvium. Except where the fever has been prolonged or recurrent, the hair loss is usually reversible.

Food Deprivation Syndrome

Noticeable hair loss may occur two to three months after a crash diet in which a person loses 15 to 20 percent of total body weight. This cause of hair loss will sometimes be missed by dermatologists who have not treated the patient on a regular basis or been informed of the recent weight loss. Blood loss, including voluntary donation, may also contribute to hair loss. In both food deprivation and blood loss, the attendant hair loss is thought to be a consequence of the reduction of proteins necessary for hair growth. In seeking medical advice about hair loss, it is important to tell the examining physician if a change in diet or blood loss has occurred. For most people who resume proper nutritional intake, the hair will begin to grow again 3 to 12 months after the acute insult.

Iron Deficiency

Even in the absence of anemia, iron deficiency may be responsible for diffuse hair loss. This is a common condition and may occur particularly in women. In fact, iron-deficiency anemia is one of the most common causes of diffuse hair loss in women, so iron levels should be tested in all women with nonscarring hair loss. Dramatic regrowth usually begins three to six months after iron supplementation is instituted.

Essential Fatty Acid Deficiency

Infants or adults on long-term supplemental, intravenous, or tube-administered nutrition may suffer hair loss because of the lack of certain fatty acids in these regimens. Preceding or accompanying the hair loss will be a dry, scaling eruption of the skin folds that resembles eczema, diffuse eyebrow and scalp hair loss, and a lightening in color of the remaining hair. Treatment includes dietary supplementation of linoleic acid or safflower oil (which is constituted of 60 to 70 percent linoleic acid). New hair growth and healing of the skin lesions follows treatment as quickly as a few weeks.

Biotin Deficiency

Biotin is an essential element in fatty acid and amino acid metabolism. A deficiency in this vitamin appears as a diffuse loss of scalp and body hair with an eczemalike scaling rash involving the mouth and torso. It can also contribute to blurred vision, gait disturbance, muscle weakness, and tremors.

The most common cause of biotin deficiency is the consumption of raw eggs, which leads to an inability of the intestine to absorb nutrients properly. The condition can also be linked to small bowel resection, nutrition delivered through a means other than the alimentary system, or a genetic, inherited deficiency. This condition responds rapidly to biotin supplementation.

Zinc Deficiency

The highest concentrations of zinc are in meat, fish, and some vegetables, although vegetables alone may not offer a sufficient source of this mineral. Zinc deficiency can be found in association with malabsorption syndromes, intravenous or tube feeding with inadequate zinc supplementation, and a genetic disease in which insufficient quantities of zinc are absorbed (acrodermatitis enteropathica).

The first indication of a zinc deficiency is diarrhea, followed by apathy, confusion, and mental depression. Abnormalities in taste and smell may also develop. In zinc deficiency states, the hair becomes fine, dry, and brittle. Eczemalike scaling eruptions on the mouth and extremities develop, followed by generalized diffuse hair loss. If a dermatologist has been consulted because of hair loss, the patient should be sure the mention other accompanying symptoms to help the physician make the proper diagnosis. Zinc supplementation has shown dramatic results, restoring the hair to its normal structure and texture.

INFECTIONS

Syphilis

Secondary or tertiary syphilis causes a characteristic "moth-eaten" scaly scalp baldness, occasionally with additional involvement of the lateral part of the eyebrows as well as of other body hair. The hair loss is patchy and often diffuse throughout the scalp.

Penicillin therapy will lead to reversal of hair loss caused by secondary syphilis. However, the destructive lesions of tertiary syphilis can lead to scarring hair loss, often irreversible despite appropriate therapy.

PREGNANCY

Although many women maintain that their hair seems especially attractive and healthy during pregnancy, hair density does not increase; in fact, the rate of hair growth is slightly reduced during pregnancy. However, during the second half of pregnancy, the percentage of active, growing hairs increases from a normal 85 percent to approximately 95 percent, and the percentage of hairs of large shaft diameter is greater than in nonpregnant women of the same age.

For some women, the hair seems sparser than normal during pregnancy. This occurs when hair follicles go into the regressed phase and cannot reenter the active, growing phase during pregnancy. This condition causes the shedding that creates the appearance of thinning hair. For others, it is only after childbirth that large numbers of follicles go into the regressed phase together.

Pregnant women and new mothers who are upset by their loss of hair should be assured that in a majority of cases almost total regrowth can be expected within a short time. Often the changes in a woman's hair are less severe during subsequent pregnancies. Inherited baldness that may be present in genetically predisposed women during pregnancy almost always reverses itself after childbirth.

∽

ENDOCRINE DISORDERS

Hypothyroidism, pituitary disorders, and parathyroid disease can all affect hair follicles.

Diffuse increased shedding of hair, loss of pigmentation from the skin *(vitiligo)*, and patchy hair loss are most commonly associated with hypothyroidism, a decrease in thyroid activity. Patients with overactive thyroid glands usually have fine, sparse hair that may occasionally be of lighter color than normal.

Patients who have underactive pituitary glands from an unknown cause or a tumor may lose scalp, underarm, and pubic hair and experience accompanying yellowness and dryness of the skin.

Parathyroid diseases have been connected with patchy hair loss.

The hair loss caused by these diseases is usually reversible with adequate treatment of the condition. Hormone replacement or suppression will often help reverse these changes, unless the disease has been so prolonged and severe that the hair follicles have become atrophied and scarred. Hair loss and change as just outlined should, therefore, not be ignored. Medical help should be sought as soon as symptoms appear.

∽

COLLAGEN VASCULAR DISEASES/VASCULITIS

Lupus (Systemic Lupus Erythematosus)

Lupus is an autoimmune defect that targets specific organs, including the skin and hair follicles. Patients usually complain about sun sensitivity (sun-induced redness), butterfly rash of the face, hair loss, arthritis, and other systemic symptoms. Dry, sparse, thin hairs on the front of the scalp (lupus hair) may be observed with this condition, and hair loss is present in approximately 50 percent of cases of acute lupus. The hair loss may be reversible with systemic anti-inflammatory or immunosuppressive therapy, such as corticosteroids or other immunosuppressive agents, for instance, Immuran or cyclosporine. The side effects—including kidney failure, high blood pressure, and liver dysfunction—must be carefully monitored.

A form of lupus that is chronic and often localized to the skin *(discoid lupus)* is sometimes accompanied by diffuse hair loss, itching, and scarring hair loss *(cicatricial alopecia)* as well as inflammatory plaques that destroy the hair follicles. Discoid lupus may be treated with topical applications or injections of corticosteroids. Antimalarial medications have also been shown to be effective for this disease.

Dermatomyositis

A rare disorder causing skin rashes and muscular weakness, *dermatomyositis*, like lupus, is thought to have an immunologic cause. During the acute stages of dermatomyositis there may be associated excessive hair growth *(hypertrichosis)*, especially on the face and extremities. Patients with this condition may also have rashes on the face, around the eyes (heliotrope), and on the extensor extremities, particularly the knuckles (Gottron's sign). Over 50 percent of people over the age of 40 who have this disease have an associated malignancy. Diffuse hair loss is present in 15 to 20 percent of cases.

With treatment, almost complete regrowth of hair is possible, although a long-term state of the disease may cause chronic scarring and hair loss. The treatments include corticosteroids, Cytoxan, and other immunosuppressive agents. The associated malignancy—if there is one—will require separate treatment.

Sjögren's Syndrome

Occurring mostly in women between the ages of 30 and 70, Sjögren's syndrome may be associated with other autoimmune disorders, such as rheumatoid arthritis, Hashimoto's thyroiditis, alopecia areata, and lupus erythematosus. Individuals who have this condition may have dry eyes and mouth (*keratoconjunctivitis sicca*), sore anogenital mucous membranes, and fine, dry, sparse hair, which can involve the pubic and axillary zones. The treatment involves immunosuppressant and anti-inflammatory therapy (discussed in the preceding section) and local therapy in the form of lubricating eye drops for the control of the dry mouth–dry eye syndrome *(sicca)*.

Giant Cell Arteritis (Temporal Arteritis)

This disease is thought to be an autoimmune disorder of the large and medium-size arteries of the elderly. Giant cell arteritis *(temporal arteritis)* results in severe headaches and muscle weakness (*polymyalgia rheumatica*) and can appear as scalp ulcerations with diffuse hair loss. In severe cases, blinding may result. The acute phase of this disease may be precipitated by overexposure to sunlight. The treatment is oral steroids, usually given in high dosages, which leads to reversal of the hair loss.

Lymphomas

Tumors such as mycoses fungoides (T cell lymphoma), Hodgkin's disease, and non-Hodgkin's lymphomas may cause firm, pink-to-brown skin-colored papules or nodules on the scalp, which can lead to scarring hair loss. Chemotherapy for the diseases may lead to reversible hair loss. When the tumors infiltrate the scalp, they are usually treated with other sites of disease, using radiation, chemotherapy, immunotherapy, or multiple modalities. The chemotherapy produces diffuse shedding of actively growing hair, which will usually totally regrow 6 to 12 months after the treatment is completed.

Chronic Liver Disease

Diffuse, progressive, nonscarring hair loss can be found with chronic liver diseases (hepatitis, cirrhoses) and iron excess diseases (hemochromatosis). It is thought that hair involvement in chronic liver disease is associated with lower protein levels in the body. The hair is often dry and breaks easily. Reproteinizing conditioners and moisturizers can help improve texture, overall appearance, and the structural integrity of the hair.

Kidney Disease

Hair loss as a result of kidney disease is particularly prominent in hemodialysis patients as a result of loss of protein and other factors. Control of the signs of uremia involving multiple organ systems is often helpful in slowing down the progression of hair loss. Such hair loss is at least partially reversible, depending on the duration and control of kidney function.

People who have chronic kidney disease may find that, as with people who suffer from chronic liver disease, their hair is dry and lusterless. The use of reproteinizing conditioners and moisturizers often helps.

6

Unwanted Hair

The gradual disappearance of body hair from the human body is the result of evolution. However, some individuals have excess body hair. This condition, called *hirsutism*, is characterized by excessive growth of terminal hair. In most cases this condition is the result of genetic variation.

Excess body hair can be embarrassing, at times to the point of trauma. Folklore and fables often portray villains as "hairy creatures," from werewolves to the big, bad wolf. The bearded woman is a circus curiosity; witches have often been portrayed as having hairy chins. In modern society, the ideal man has body hair only on his chest and legs. The ideal woman, as created by current advertisements, doesn't have any excess body hair at all.

The majority of men who do have excess body hair on their backs or shoulders appear to be psychologically able to handle the situation. Women, however, are extremely sensitive to excess body hair. Hirsute women can feel freakish and dirty. Some fear that their sexual identity is threatened, the excess hair suggesting masculinity.

The fact is that all normal women have hair over most of their bodies. However, this covering is usually made up of virtually invisible vellus hair. A report in the British medical journal *Lancet* surveyed the amount of body hair in normal young British women and found that 26 percent had facial hair, 17 percent had hair on their chests or breasts, and 35 percent had lower abdominal hair. These figures have been supported by other studies. Some women, nevertheless, do have excess hair that is darker and more noticeable than average. Hirsutism can be classified into four types:

1. familial
2. idiopathic
3. drug induced
4. hormonal (androgen excess)

Although the cause or causes are not always readily detected, hirsutism can result from a variety of factors. Certain medical procedures and tests can help find the causes. It is most important to determine whether excess hair is a normal genetic variation or a sign of an underlying pathological disease.

It is possible for a woman to be hairy simply because of a family history of this condition, with no significant underlying disease. Sometimes, the source of the hirsutism cannot be readily detected at all and must be accepted as a normal variable characteristic trait for that person. However, the majority of hirsute women have increased androgen production, derived from either the ovaries or the adrenal glands (the two major endocrinologic glands in women responsible for the production of androgen hormones) or from increased sensitivity of the hair follicles to these masculinizing hormones.

∽

HIRSUTISM RELATED TO ANDROGEN EXCESS

Increased androgen production results in increased hair growth, changed pigmentation of the hair, larger diameter of the hair shaft, and the conversion of fine vellus hair to thick terminal hair, all of which make the hair more prominent and visible.

There are ovarian and adrenal function tests to help discover if hormone imbalance is causing the excess hair growth. These tests should be performed on all women who have excessive growth of coarse terminal body hair in a male growth pattern, particularly if there is no family history of this condition. These tests may be classified into blood hormone measurements and stimulatory and suppressive tests of glandular function.

The major hormones to be tested include

1. testosterone
2. DHEAS (dihydroepiandrosterone-sulfate), an androgen metabolite
3. sex hormone binding globulin, a protein that "binds" to androgens
4. Prolactin, a hormone produced by the pituitary gland and associated with the production of breast milk, menstrual abnormalities, and the inability to conceive. It

also may be associated with polycystic ovary syndrome.

Other hormone tests include those of the LH/FSH (luteinizing hormone/follicle-stimulating hormone) ratio. These stimulatory hormones regulate ovarian and, subsequently, menstrual function.

More sophisticated tests of adrenal functions include stimulatory (ACTH stimulation) and suppressive (dexamethasone suppression) endocrine evaluations. In addition, measurements of urinary steroid metabolites may be elevated in androgen-excess syndromes responsible for hirsutism.

Once the cause of the condition is ascertained, there are effective treatments, although most have side effects that must be carefully monitored.

If an androgen excess is discovered, the primary therapy is the use of antiandrogens, drugs that suppress terminal hair growth. Antiandrogen medications include cyproterone acetate, a potent progestational derivative that suppresses terminal hair growth. Cyproterone acetate has been successfully used in the treatment of hirsutism, acne, and seborrhea in Europe but is not available for general use in the United States because of its unpleasant side effects, such as weight gain, depression, and loss of libido. Moreover, use must be accompanied by birth control therapy because the medication may cause feminization (development of female sexual characteristics) of a male fetus. This treatment, while effective, is not recommended.

Another antiandrogen is spironolactone (Aldactone), an anti–high blood pressure drug, that acts in two important ways: It inhibits androgen biosynthesis and inhibits androgen receptors formed in the hair follicle. Spironolactone is available in the United States. The major side effect of this medication is that it causes menstrual irregularities.

Cimetidine is a more controversial drug. Used primarily as an antiulcer medication (it is an H2 antihistamine), it also acts as an antiandrogen. The efficacy of this drug in the treatment of hirsutism is questionable.

A new treatment, flutamide, in combination with oral contraceptive therapy, is one of the strongest antiandrogens. It shows promise but is still being tested in the United States for the treatment of hirsutism.

If adrenal gland overactivity is noted, low-dose bedtime corticosteroid therapy may be instituted. Close patient monitoring is essential to avoid potential serious side effects of chronic steroid usage, including diabetes, high blood pressure, bone abnormalities of the hip, mood changes, and gastrointestinal upset.

It is important to note that although there are drugs that can be effective, all of them have drawbacks. Treatments take three to four months before there is any recycling of existing terminal hair. And no matter what drug treatment is used, the patient must still often remove a certain amount of hair physically because no drug completely suppresses terminal hair growth.

Further medical and gynecologic evaluations are required for women if one of several conditions is present. Normal hirsutism is usually a gradual progression. The excess hair growth develops slowly from puberty until the early twenties, when it reaches its final stage. If, however, the progression of hirsutism changes suddenly, there could be more serious underlying causes.

Hirsutism may be a manifestation of virilization (masculinization). Other features of this condition include deepening of the voice, decrease in breast size, enlarged genitalia, increased musculature, balding of the scalp, and late onset of severe acne or seborrhea. Combined with these developments, hirsutism can indicate the onset of virilization. The patient in this instance should have more significant evaluation to rule out potentially life-threatening conditions that may be surgically curable. This is especially so if there is severe terminal hair growth over the upper back and shoulder area.

There are also ovarian, adrenal, and pituitary conditions that can contribute to hirsutism. Ovarian tumors and even pregnancy are common contributing causes. Hirsutism caused by irregularity of the menstrual cycle may be a sign of polycystic ovarian syndrome (PCO) or prolactin-secreting tumors of the pituitary gland.

Doctors can use a number of methods to determine the presence of serious ovarian, adrenal, pituitary, or hypothalamic pathology. These include skull X rays, ultrasound, CAT scans, magnetic resonance imaging (MRI), direct adrenal sampling of blood hormone levels, and gynecologic and endocrinologic evaluations.

Drug-Induced Hirsutism

Hirsutism can also be caused by drugs, including high-progesterone birth control pills, testosterone (male hormone), minoxidil (anti–high blood pressure medication), Dilantin (antiseizure medication), steroid medications, psoralens (DNA binding agent used in conjunction with long-wave ultraviolet light to treat psoriasis), cyclosporine (immune modulatory medicine), penicillamine (metal-chelating, anti-inflammatory medication), and chlorobenzene (hydrocarbon).

HYPERTRICHOSIS

There are a number of difficulties in establishing a clear description of *hypertrichosis*. First, clinical descriptions of the pattern of hair growth are often inaccurate. Second, it differs from hirsutism, with which it is often confused, in that hair growth is not hormone dependent and occurs in unusual areas. And, third, the mechanisms controlling hair growth are poorly understood.

Both men and women can suffer from this relatively rare condition, and it can be triggered by a variety of causes.

For clarity, we classify hypertrichosis by whether it has a congenital or an acquired cause.

Congenital Hypertrichosis

Congenital hypertrichosis results from a chromosome that causes children to be excessively hairy at birth and to retain this hair throughout life. At times the entire skin, except palms and soles of the feet, may be covered by fine, silky hair as long as 4 inches.

This disease can accompany congenital moles (Becker's melanosis) or may be associated with areas of irregularity of the central nervous system, particularly structural abnormalities of the spinal cord such as spina bifida, which is a developmental abnormality of the spinal cord. Other congenital hypertrichosis syndromes may be associated with certain neurological disorders.

Congenital hypertrichosis may also be associated with various metabolic disorders (lipoatrophic diabetes, Lawrence Siep syndrome, Cornelia de Lange's syndrome, Rubinstein-Taybi syndrome); disorders of connective tissue (Winchester syndrome); abnormalities of red blood cell enzyme function (posphyrias); malnutrition; and anorexia nervosa (an eating disorder). Pregnant women who ingest alcohol or the anticonvulsant drug Dilantin may also be affected. Severe emaciation may result in patients who have downy hypertrichosis of the trunk and arms. Underactive thyroid function (hypothyroidism) may also be associated with hypertrichosis.

Acquired Hypertrichosis

Acquired hypertrichosis may indicate an underlying malignancy or may occur after head injuries or other cerebral disturbances, usually one to four months after the injury. Spontaneous recovery is the rule. In such a situation, the mechanism for the growth of excess hair is unknown.

When treating excess hair caused by an identified medical condition, the rule is to treat the underlying condition rather than focus on this one symptom.

ℭ

REMOVING EXCESS HAIR

There are essentially eight methods of removing excess hair. Because people react differently to the various procedures, each person needs to find the procedure that works best, causes the least irritation, and lasts longest with the least serious side effects for him or her.

Shaving

Perhaps the oldest known method of removing excess hair is shaving. Many women regularly shave their legs with an electric razor. However, electric razors cannot cut the hair as closely as a blade, and the rough stubble often left by an electric razor can be as objectionable to touch as the hair was to see. But the electric razor is safer because with it the possibility of cutting the skin is eliminated.

Wet shaving with a safety razor and cream allows the hair to be cut closely at the skin's surface. But problems exist with this procedure as well. For example, many women suffer skin irritation when they use a blade. Also, blade shaving can help spread infections such as impetigo, viral warts, and herpes simplex, or cause ingrown hairs. This is why it is important to avoid using other people's personal care items and to clean those you use. Shaving with either a blade or an electric razor is not recommended for underarms, where regrowing hair shafts may cause irritation or secondary infection of the hair follicles. And shaving may be particularly uncomfortable and cause inflammation of the hair follicles in the pubic area. Incidentally, there is little scientific evidence to support the popular belief that shaving increases either coarse hair texture or subsequent hair growth.

Depilatories

Chemical depilatory agents dissolve the hair shaft by reducing the disulfide bonds within it. The primary ingredient in these preparations is calcium thioglycolate, although some also contain sulfur compounds of calcium, arsenic, antimony, barium, and strontium in a cream base. The compounds reduce the hair to a jellylike consistency, which can be wiped off the skin. A good moisturizer or calamine lotion will help soothe redness or irritation caused by the procedure, but some people have uncomfortable allergic reactions to depilatories. Furthermore, the moisturizers may also cause allergic reactions, leading to skin irritation.

It is mandatory that patch-testing be done before the use of a depilatory cream to be sure that a person is not allergic to its ingredients. A 24-hour test should be done on the inside of the wrist. If irritation is noted at the patch site, the product should not be used.

Aside from a possible allergic reaction, the main disadvantages of depilatory creams are that they are expensive and must be used repeatedly.

Bleaching

Bleaching excess hair removes the natural hair pigment, thus making hair less noticeable. Four types of commercial hair bleaches whose active ingredient is hydrogen peroxide are available: neutral oil bleaches, color oil bleaches, cream bleaches, and powder bleaches. These agents produce varying degrees of bleaching. It should be noted that bleaching agents can cause occasional local irritation.

Gloves

Hair-removing gloves are mittens made of fine sandpaper. More popular in Europe than in the United States, the gloves are rubbed in a circular motion to remove stubble from areas of the body.

Tweezing

Tweezing is effective because the plucking action removes the complete hair shaft, thus providing a longer period before the hair regrows. There is little skin damage associated with tweezing hair. The process is, however, tedious and mildly uncomfortable, and consequently really not feasible for large areas.

Waxing

Hair waxing is actually a variation of tweezing. There are two methods, hot and cold waxing. Hot waxing is accomplished by applying beeswax or another low-melting-point wax to the hair. Once the wax has set, it is pulled away, taking with it the trapped hairs down the level of the hair bulb. Waxing may induce skin irritation and, occasionally, inflammation of the hair follicle. Obviously, the main side effect of hot waxing is burning. Another disadvantage of waxing is that the hairs have to be at least ⅟₁₆ inch in length before the wax can grip them sufficiently to remove them. This problem can be minimized by waxing different areas at different times and bleaching between waxings.

Cold waxing utilizes a wax that is squeezed as a liquid from a pouch. It is applied to a cloth that covers the area to be treated. When the cloth is removed, the wax comes with it. This is an excellent method of hair removal because the cloth can be taken off as one piece, rather than in bits, as in hot waxing. Cold waxing also removes both coarse and fine hairs, which makes it very functional for the upper lip, chin, eyebrows, and cheeks of women. Men rarely find facial cold waxing acceptable, because of the cumbersome technique.

In general the waxing process must be repeated at intervals ranging between two and six weeks. Waxing can cause local irritation.

Epilating

Epilating is a mechanized method of plucking hair. The apparatus used contains a tightly coiled spring that traps hair and pulls it out at the level of the hair bulb. Despite advertisements to the contrary, there are some problems with these tools. Epilating can be painful and is particularly uncomfortable on areas of the body where the skin is thin, such as the face. This method's effectiveness is also severely limited on curved surfaces, such as the underarms. Because there is significant manipulation of the hair follicle, infection and skin trauma are often major side effects of this kind of treatment. These adverse consequences can be minimized by the use of topical aseptic detergents, soaps, and topical antibiotics. Also, a 1 to 2 percent hydrocortisone preparation is sometimes helpful in reducing skin redness.

Electrolysis

Electrolysis is the only potentially permanent method of removing hair. The process utilizes a small needle, which is inserted into the hair follicle. An electric current sent through the needle to the hair shaft destroys the follicle. After the needle is withdrawn, the hair is removed with a forceps. Although electrolysis is considered a permanent hair-removal process, regrowth ranging from 15 to 50 percent of the hair removed can occur.

Electrolysis can cause scarring at the site of removal, particularly if poor technique is employed. Other problems associated with electrolysis include the onset of acne-type eruptions and the precipitation of active herpes simplex infection. There is also some risk of contracting hepatitis or AIDS through unsterile equipment or careless procedures. It should also be noted that electrolysis is less successful when androgen excess is inducing the unusual growth. Time and expense may be saved if electrolysis is deferred until hormone therapy has slowed the appearance of new hair. This procedure must be performed by an experienced, board-certified technician called an electrologist.

PART THREE

TREATMENTS
for
HAIR
LOSS

7

Unproven Treatments for Hair Loss

It would seem to be really very easy to find a cure for baldness. After all, there are dozens of "experts" ready to sell nutritional, herbal, or vitamin breakthroughs guaranteed to provide a full head of hair.

Banking on the balding person's tendency to try virtually anything to get his or her hair back is not a contemporary phenomenon. Throughout history people have been looking for a quick, easy method of growing lost hair. According to Herodotus (c. 484–425 B.C.), the Egyptians had a "physician of the head," who specialized in diseases of the scalp; one Egyptian remedy for baldness instructed men to rub their scalps vigorously with a concoction of dates, dogs' paws, and asses' hooves ground up and cooked together. Another surefire remedy required equal parts of fat from a lion, a hippopotamus, a crocodile, a goose, a snake, and an ibex to be applied liberally to the scalp. Cleopatra attempted to cure Julius Caesar's baldness with burned domestic mice, horse teeth, bear grease, and deer marrow.

In the late 1600s various combinations of myr-
tle leaves, pine tree bark, white wine, oil of radish
seed, sorrel, myrrh, willow leaves, oil of green
grapes, juniper berries, wormwood, fern roots, lin-
seed oil, bruised almonds, wheat bran, and master
powder (natural hair growth–promoting concoctions) were considered great hair-growing preparations.

⌐ Because product regulation around the world is
less stringent than in the United States, a great many
countries have produced and are still producing
some interesting baldness "cures." For example, in
France a mixture of rum alcohol, beef marrow, and
bergamot oil is claimed to grow hair. People in the
Soviet Union maintain they have cured baldness
with acupuncture. West Germany offers extract of
fresh bovine heart and lecithin to stimulate hair
growth. Some people in Hungary mix horseradish,
mustard oil, orange and lemon peel, and egg yolk.
Hungarian experts say that this combination accel-
erates keratin formation by the hair bulbs, noting a
"cure" rate of 44 percent in just 12 weeks. In Japan,
hair is said to "sprout" after treatment with vitamin
E, vitamin B_2, gibberellin, and papain. Another recommended treatment is administered with a "special" brush. A person is instructed to hit himself or
herself 200 times daily, in order to increase blood
flow and thus stimulate hair growth.

It is also possible to find some rather unusual,
and medically unproven, methods of growing hair in
the United States. Among the most bizarre is a "surefire" method based on folklore. According to believ-
ers, allowing (perhaps persuading) a cow to lick the
head of a bald man will cause hair to grow, presum-
ably on the man's head, not the cow's tongue. And,

despite the fact that this idea is not taken seriously by anyone in the medical community, it has been discovered that cattle saliva contains a substance that promotes the growth of skin and its appendages, including hair. But it doesn't make hair grow on people.

It isn't just peculiar concoctions that give hope to the hairless. Some have suggested that raw, fresh vegetables and low-fat protein foods can decrease hair loss. Another recipe includes six glasses of water a day and avoidance of animal fat and foods containing vitamin B. Others claim that removing salt from the diet will encourage hair to grow.

Additional remedies include massage (executed with hand vibrators), which some feel increases blood flow to the scalp and thus heightens the supply of oxygen and nutrients to the hair. Hair popping, another so-called remedy, is accomplished by a high-frequency machine. The patient holds a heated rod called a saturator, which passes an electric current through his or her body. When the machine's operator touches the patient's scalp, an electric circuit is completed and the patient receives a kind of pins-and-needles sensation. Likewise, when the operator yanks the patient's hair, an electric circuit is completed and a mild shock, the popping, results. Although massage and popping may increase the blood circulation in the scalp, neither has ever been shown to increase hair growth.

There is even a theory that shaving the head is good for the hair and scalp. Some men believe that if they frequently shave their heads the hair will come back thicker, coarser, and more abundant. This is just not true.

In fact, none of these procedures has been

either medically or scientifically proven to be effective. Most cost a lot and are offered with supreme confidence. They are all, however, triumphs of hope over reality.

It can be flatly stated that no over-the-counter formulations or devices have been proven to grow hair on a bald scalp, and no precise method for assessing hair growth has been established.

The Food and Drug Administration (FDA) has publicly specified that products claiming to prevent baldness or stimulate hair growth are "not generally recognized as safe and effective," and there are laws designed to prevent the sale of these preparations. However, these laws are not always effective. For one thing, it has been found that if a procedure stimulates the scalp, the scalp occasionally produces downy, almost invisible vellus hair. This is, of course, not "real" hair. But, it is hair of a sort, making it difficult to prosecute the manufacturer. Also, a balding man can see the slightest increase in fuzziness as the first step to a full head of hair. And, finally, although the FDA, together with the Federal Trade Commission, has taken action against fraudulent claims, fake devices, and drugs, it has largely abandoned this enforcement tool because of the time and money necessary to bring criminal prosecutions. The agency now relies instead on public education and civil actions to deter fraud.

It is difficult for the medical profession, armed only with boring facts, to fight the persuasive techniques of swindlers, who often have impressive people, sometimes even scientists, give personal testimony about the benefits of fraudulent remedies.

8

Seeking Professional Help

A number of curious scientists and philosophers have studied hair loss as an indication of other physical abnormalities. Giambattista della Porta (1535–1615), Italian playwright, philosopher, and scientist, studied character and psychology through the contours of the head and the condition of the hair. In the famous "Aphorisms" of Hippocrates, annotated by Galen, the importance of hair loss as a symptom of other disorders is emphasized. And according to Nigel Nicolson in *Napoleon 1812*, after Napoleon invaded Russia with 500,000 troops and retreated with a mere 41,000, his chief surgeon, Baron Larrey, concluded that the bald men were the first to die from exposure to severe weather.

∾

THE DOCTOR

Modern doctors took little interest in disorders of the hair, apart from ringworm and patchy baldness, until the twentieth century, when the development of the field of endocrinology began to provide some understanding of the mechanisms underlying common disturbances of hair growth. Even today patients with no complaints about their hair or scalp rarely expect hair to be part of a regular medical checkup.

But recent research has greatly increased the medical community's knowledge of the complex endocrine influences on the hair. It has been established that a wide range of metabolic and nutritional disturbances, and some psychiatric states, may first be clinically manifested as, or accompanied by, changes in the density, pattern, color, or texture of the hair. In fact, apart from male pattern baldness and abnormalities of the hair resulting from direct infection or chemical or physical trauma to the hair, almost all changes in hair growth and condition can be directly related to another disease process. Consequently, today the wise family practitioner will routinely investigate the condition of patients' hair.

Only fully qualified medical doctors can diagnose serious hair disorders and rule out established medical causes of hair loss. It is naturally possible for any qualified medical doctor to treat simple, non-complicated scalp problems such as dandruff. But, for intensive treatment of the hair and scalp, an individual will most likely want to consult a dermatologist.

All dermatologists are trained in the care of skin and hair. However, not all dermatologists concentrate on hair and scalp problems. Some doctors consider taking care of patients who are suffering from hair loss a bother; others may restrict their practices to skin problems or particular areas of their field, such as cancer or surgery. The physician who is interested in and has studied hair-loss problems is most likely to be in touch with the newest therapeutic modalities.

To choose a physician, call a local university or community hospital and consult either the dermatology division or physicians' referral service. It is important to request a *board-certified* dermatologist, to be assured that the physician has received training in the diagnosis and treatment of hair disorders.

When making your initial appointment with any physician, describe the problem to a member of the office staff. This explanation will help assure that the doctor is, in fact, a specialist in hair loss and will save you a consultation fee if he or she is not.

Of course, even if you find a doctor who treats hair problems, additional consultations may be required. If the dermatologist finds certain symptoms, he or she will refer the patient to a secondary specialist, an endocrinologist for evaluation of possible related hormonal problems (thyroid, adrenal, and so on), a gynecologist for ovarian or contraceptive-related pathology, or an internist for evaluation of underlying medical problems (iron-deficiency anemia, drug-related alopecia, and so on).

If an individual's hair loss results from hereditary male pattern baldness, and he or she is looking for surgical corrections such as hair transplants and/or scalp reduction, it is vital to make this clear at the initial meeting. Hair transplants may be performed by dermatologic surgeons, plastic surgeons, and, occasionally, general surgeons.

Avoid trichologists. Too often desperate individuals suffering hair loss fall prey to the glossy and persuasive advertising of individuals who claim to be "experts" in hair growth. In fact, trichologists are not licensed medical doctors, and their therapeutic procedures rarely are scientifically proven or offer any scientific efficacy.

∽

THE EXAMINATION

The evaluation of a patient with hair loss must be thorough and include a careful history, good physical examination, and appropriate laboratory studies. These procedures will inform the doctor about the duration and location of the hair problems and the patient's life changes, physical development, and drug intake as well as provide familiarity with the patient's hair-care habits.

The patient should expect the doctor to examine all hair-bearing areas of the body; inspect the type and texture of hair in all areas and the pattern and distribution of hair loss; look for signs of inflammation, infection, scarring, or other cutaneous or systemic diseases; and generally evaluate his or her mental status. The complete examination is important because increased or decreased hair development as well as changing hair must be investigated. For example, increased amounts of terminal hair growing where vellus hair should be may be a sign of endocrinologic dysfunction.

Several evaluations may be performed in the

physician's office. These include a hair-pull test, in which the physician will lightly pull on 8 to 10 clustered hairs using a mechanical traction instrument. Normally 0 to 2 hairs are pulled out. If excessive shedding is present, 4 to 6 hairs are easily removed. Excessive hair easily plucked is a sign of telogen effluvium and, if this occurs around patches of baldness, the hair loss is probably a progressive disorder and likely to extend to larger areas.

Microscopic evaluation of the hair *(trichogram)* will detect hair shaft abnormalities or fungal infections, distinguish hair loss secondary to trauma or various types of drug-induced hair loss, and evaluate the percentage of hairs in the resting or growing phase.

A scalp biopsy may be indicated. This procedure may distinguish inflammatory, automechanical, and immunologic causes of hair loss, which are reversible, from the more common male pattern baldness, which is not.

∽

LABORATORY EVALUATION

A laboratory evaluation that includes hair analyses and blood tests is important to rule out endocrine conditions such as thyroid, ovarian, adrenal, hypothalamic, or pituitary disease. The blood tests will also evaluate thyroid function, testosterone and its metabolites, prolactin, pituitary stimulating hormones, and luteinizing hormone to follicle-stimulating hormone (LH/FSH) ratio. A blood chemistry profile will detect any underlying internal diseases, particularly those involving the kidneys or liver.

Not only to ensure proper treatment for hair and scalp problems but also because many systemic diseases first appear on the scalp, a patient should first find a competent, certified physician and expect, or request, a complete examination of the problem.

9

Treatments for Male Pattern Baldness

Despite the fact that much of the fascination surrounding hair-growth products appears to center on the certainly peculiar and almost inevitably useless products and procedures touted by enterprising individuals, there have been some interesting and encouraging scientific advances in treatment for male pattern baldness. For example, there seems to be hope in the study of antiandrogens. These treatments are likely to be effective for five reasons:

1. Male pattern baldness is androgen dependent. Androgens are male hormones that are believed to play a role in the distribution of body hair and the development of genetic hair loss.

Dihydrotestosterone (DHT) is the androgen responsible for hair growth over much of the body after puberty and for male pattern baldness. Balding men have increased levels of the enzyme 5 alpha reductase in the hair follicles and skin of the frontal scalp. Moreover, in certain individuals, the hair follicles are more sensitive to the activity of circulating hormones. The connection between male pattern baldness and the action of circulating hormones is supported by the discovery that men with 5 alpha reductase deficiency have sparse androgen-dependent body hairs and *do not* develop baldness.

It is also important to note that increased androgen production, sensitivity of the scalp to androgens, and conversion of androgen metabolites by means of increased enzyme activity appear to be important in the development of male pattern baldness in women. The condition is normally less common and severe in women simply because their androgen levels are lower. Women who experience the onset of male pattern baldness before menopause usually have a history of baldness in male family members as well as other signs of excess androgens, such as acne or hirsutism. Baldness in women may also be a manifestation of congenital adrenal hyperplasia, Cushing's disease, or androgen-producing tumors. However, most often no serious underlying abnormality is discovered.

2. Scientific observations demonstrate that men castrated before puberty do not have any circulating male hormones and consequently do not develop baldness.

3. If castrated men are given androgens, baldness may ensue.

4. Scalp hair thinning is arrested in men who are castrated after puberty, but little or no regrowth occurs.

5. Further hair loss may be prevented with

antiandrogens, but substantial regrowth of scalp hair is unlikely to occur with these agents alone.

In both sexes, it is clear that androgens play if not the complete then certainly a major role in baldness.

Antiandrogens are substances that inhibit the biological function of androgenic hormones. They may block the effect of these hormones by competitively binding to receptor sites where they produce their biological action, or inhibit enzymes that are necessary for the hormones to function actively. Oral antiandrogens have been shown to be effective in the treatment of male pattern baldness in women. In men, however, oral treatment with these preparations has been shown to cause loss of libido, impotence, and growth of breasts *(gynecomastia)*.

TOPICAL PREPARATIONS

To avoid the side effects caused by oral antiandrogen therapy, some men have been treated with topical preparations. High concentrations of these agents used on the balding scalp show hope but have not yet been proven totally effective.

Progesterone is an inhibitor of 5 alpha reductase. It has been widely used as a topical antiandrogen. Anecdotal reports and uncontrolled studies have yielded mixed results, because progesterone does not stay in place long enough to do much good. It is rapidly metabolized and unlikely to remain active for long.

Topical estrogen therapy has also shown mixed results in combating hair loss. Estrogen acts as an antagonist on the male androgenic hormone. Because of its side effect of increased breast size, this is not a particularly encouraging treatment.

Cyproterone acetate, an antiandrogen drug administered orally, has been shown to be effective in the treatment of male pattern baldness in women but ineffective for men. Consequently, this substance has been used topically and by injection on men. However, so far, the results have been equivocal. The drug has not yet been approved for use in this country and is not recommended at this time.

Spironolactone, a diuretic (water pill) with androgen receptor antagonist properties, has been studied as a topical preparation with conflicting results.

Cyoctol is a nonsteroidal compound that inhibits androgen binding to DHT receptors in skin cells. In the spring of 1990, researchers found that this drug seems to halt hair loss and, to a certain degree, increase hair growth in men with male pattern baldness. A study by Chantel, the Los Angeles–based pharmaceutical firm that developed the drug, showed that of 12 men using a 0.5 percent solution for 48 weeks, 10 increased their hair counts by 3 percent; 5 of 9 men using a 0.1 percent formula showed an increased growth of 4 percent.

Cyoctol has not, however, proven to be a magic potion. Critics point out that more than half of the original study group fell out before the research was over, and many investigators feel that the drug has not proven effective at truly preventing or slowing hair loss, or at stimulating its regrowth. Although

Bristol-Myers–Squibb originally acquired the rights to develop and market Cyoctol, it has returned those rights to Chantel. Also, the drug has not been approved by the FDA because of its questionable efficacy. Upjohn has acquired rights to this drug and plans further clinical studies.

However, some scientists feel that, after further studies, Cyoctol will help prevent hair loss in some women who have a history of baldness in their families. If this drug actually prevents the balding process from beginning, it would have an edge over minoxidil, which is effective only after hair loss has begun. This drug is still experimental and the side effects are not known. It is not recommended at this time.

∽

SYSTEMIC PREPARATIONS

For Women

Along with topical solutions and drugs, several systemic preparations to treat hair loss are being tested.

Cyproterone acetate is a potent antiandrogen progestational agent. It suppresses pituitary activity as well as interferes with androgen binding with the receptors of the hair follicle. In addition to its value in the treatment of hair loss, cyproterone acetate is helpful for hirsutism, acne, and dandruff. So far there has been little scientific evidence of regrowth of hair in women using this drug, but doses of 50 to 100 milligrams a day combined with ethinyl estradiol to induce menstruation may prevent further

progression of hair loss. Conditions that contraindi-
cate the use of this drug include cigarette smoking,
obesity, and hypertension. The side effects of cyproterone acetate include weight gain, fatigue, loss of
libido, nausea, headaches, and depression. Because
of these side effects, this drug is not available in the
United States. Use of this drug is not recommended
at this time.

Spironolactone is a potent antiandrogen with an
affinity for human androgen receptors. By binding to
these receptors, it acts as an antagonist to testosterone.

This drug appears to be the best currently available treatment for androgen-induced hair loss in
women. Side effects such as nausea, fatigue, head-
ache, and irregular menses are common with high
doses (150 to 400 mg a day), but lower doses (50 to
100 mg a day) are generally well tolerated. The drug
can prevent masculinization of the male fetus, so
patients cannot be or get pregnant while using spironolactone. It also can increase the frequency of
menses and elevate potassium levels, which can be
dangerous to patients with kidney disease. This drug
is not approved for use in the United States by the
FDA and is not recommended for use at this time.

Cyclic estrogen therapy has been used for both
adrenal and ovarian androgen hyperactivity but is
most helpful in ovarian androgen excess. Estrogen
combinations, such as Norgestrel and Levonorges-
trel, are used. The preferred cyclic estrogens are
Demulen, Ortho-Novum, and Ovcon. These are most
helpful for women in whom elevated androgens of
ovarian or adrenal origin are responsible for hair
loss. These agents inhibit the action of androgens.

Cimetidine is an antihistamine of the H2 receptor type as well as a weak antiandrogen. Although initial studies of this drug show promising results on hirsutism (androgens may produce excessive hair growth and hirsutism as well as alopecia), there are no good, double-blind, controlled studies of its use in the treatment of male pattern baldness.

For Men

Finasteride (Proscar) is a steroid inhibitor of 5 alpha reductase. Laboratory studies indicate that finasteride may be the most potent antiandrogen therapy for male pattern baldness. It may prevent progression of male pattern thinning and has been shown to stop the progression of baldness in animals.

There are studies in progress to determine the effect of orally administered finasteride on the scalp skin of men with male pattern baldness. These studies have also been valuable in supporting the concept that local 5 alpha reductase inhibitors play an important role in male pattern baldness.

Antiandrogen therapy for male pattern baldness is in its infancy. It is clear that, for men, topical antiandrogens hold the most promise because of the side effects that result from systemic administration of the currently available drugs. For women, systemic antiandrogens appear to be a responsible option, producing good subjective results. However, despite the promising data, further research is needed to document the long-term risks and efficacy of systemic antiandrogen therapy in women.

10

New Biological Modifiers for Hair Growth

A *biological modifier* is an agent that produces a given effect by altering the physiological regulation of an organ system, in this case hair. Several biological modifiers have been, and are being, studied as possible hair-growth treatments.

∽
MINOXIDIL

The first indications that minoxidil, a drug used to control high blood pressure, had some effect on hair growth came in 1980, when a researcher reported hair regrowth in a patient following the use of oral minoxidil for hypertension. Moreover, 80 percent of those taking Loniten tablets (which contain minoxidil) for high blood pressure experienced hair growth during initial utilization. These reports naturally created a stir and almost immediate further investigation into the possible use of minoxidil to treat male pattern baldness as well as patchy baldness.

It was quickly determined that taking the drug orally was not a good idea for anyone not suffering from high blood pressure because of the possible serious side effects, such as rapid heart rate, fainting, vomiting, difficulty in breathing, and accumulation of fluid around the heart. Consequently, researchers began testing compounded minoxidil in a topical solution and instructed balding men to rub it into their scalps. These studies indicated that minoxidil is capable of inducing variable degrees of mature, pigmented hair regrowth in both male pattern baldness and secondary nonscarring baldness resulting from trauma.

The mechanism of action for minoxidil is not totally understood, although several hypotheses have been offered. The drug appears to cause an enlargement of the hair follicle by extending the active growth cycle. In addition, investigators have demonstrated that the drug induces a localized immunologic change around the hair follicle, increases blood flow to the hair matrix, inhibits the activities of connective tissue cells (fibroblasts) that produce the structural building blocks of the skin, and is a potassium channel antagonist, interfering with the active metabolic regulation of the hair follicle. The precise mechanism for the hair-growth-promoting action of minoxidil remains unknown, and a receptor site in the follicle has yet to be discovered. However, it is felt that, in order to reverse male pattern baldness, topical minoxidil must continuously oppose the normal genetic program in the balding area.

But just how effective is it? Most of the data concerning the effectiveness of minoxidil come from the 27-center clinical trial run by the Upjohn Company. The double-blind, randomized trials tested the effect of topical minoxidil on men with male pattern baldness. Efficacy was measured by hair growth, investigators' evaluations, and patient evaluations. The study demonstrated that Upjohn's product Rogaine was safe and effective for male pattern baldness of the crown and would reverse, at least partially, follicular miniaturization.

However, critics point out that the clinical studies were anecdotal, the reports were potentially biased, open labeled (that is, which patients were using minoxidil and which were using a placebo was not kept secret in some cases), uncontrolled, and subjective. In addition, the study is criticized because of the limited duration of the placebo phase of the tests, inconsistent hair counting, and lack of standardization of photographic technique.

The most effective dose is also still being studied. Minoxidil is available in a 2 percent solution from the Upjohn Company. However, dermatologists have used preparations with up to 5 percent. It is felt that, in concentrations up to 5 percent, systemic absorption of the drug is minimal. But with a 7.5 percent concentration, minoxidil has been noted to cause unwarranted side effects.

The use of topical minoxidil within the guidelines of the Upjohn-sponsored study was shown to be safe. However, participants in their investigations were carefully selected, healthy, motivated, and perhaps more informed than the routine patient about male pattern baldness. Minoxidil does not cause abnormalities of the chromosomes, cancer, or birth defects. The drug is eliminated from body tissue within four days.

Since being released from Canada in 1986, Rogaine has had a good safety profile, with only 2 percent of 24,500 patients using the drug having any adverse reaction. None of these reactions has been severe; most involve inflammation on the scalp. However, patients over the age of 50, those with systemic disease, those with scalp abnormalities (which could lead to increased absorption of the drug), and anyone taking medicines that may interact adversely with minoxidil naturally require special attention.

On average, of any group of patients using the drug, one-third grow hair that is visible, one-third grow vellus hair, and one-third experience no growth at all. However, 70 to 90 percent of patients experience stabilization of their remaining hair. Optimistic results have also been reported in females with androgenetic hair loss. Nevertheless, it is rare to realize prebalding hair density with the use of minoxidil. Hair structure is often somewhat wispy and occasionally has decreased pigmentation.

Initial studies indicate that posterior hair loss seems to respond best to minoxidil. Anterior hairline baldness does not seem to respond as well as baldness on the top, or crown. It also appears that younger patients, those with smaller areas of baldness, and those with at least 100 mature or intermediate hairs in a 1-inch balding area have the best chances of success with minoxidil treatment. Minoxidil has recently been approved by the FDA for use in women with male pattern baldness. Early reports indicate that it may be more effective in women with this kind of hair loss than in men.

Hair regrowth does not happen quickly. With twice-daily applications, new hair growth can take at least 4 months, and the treatment may have to continue for up to 12 months before any new hair is apparent. Even then, in most patients the results are subtle and consist of barely perceptible vellus hairs. It must also be stressed that if topical use of minoxidil is discontinued, the scalp reverts toward its baseline state, and increased hair loss and further progression of male pattern baldness are noted within 2 to 3 months. In other words, use of minoxidil is a lifetime commitment. And it is not cheap. Currently treatment with minoxidil costs between $50 and $100 a month, depending on the concentration utilized.

Nevertheless, minoxidil clearly does work on some people, in some areas of hair loss, at some times. The ultimate reputation of the drug depends on a realistic appraisal of patient expectations. Most balding men want to see hair, not fuzz. And, at the present time, minoxidil alone does not seem to be the final answer. Upjohn's appraisal of Rogaine's effectiveness seems overly optimistic. However, future studies may find that it can be successfully employed with other drugs.

There are reports that using a combination of topical minoxidil and 0.025 percent trentoin (Retin solution) can be helpful in enhancing hair growth. And minoxidil is being used with retinoic acid, which also may have intrinsic hair-growth-promoting qualities. Minoxidil and retinoic acid should be applied separately; mixing these agents may interfere with the clinical activity of each. Both may cause local irritations.

It is important to keep in mind that minoxidil has been approved by the FDA (it is one of the few hair-growing drugs to receive this distinction), and research on the drug continues. Currently, minoxidil is available commercially only in a 2 percent concentration, but, as noted, studies are being done on 3 to 5 percent solutions. In addition, new analogues of minoxidil, with increased hair-growth-promoting activities, are being investigated.

DIAZOXIDE

Diazoxide is another drug currently being studied. This is a sugar-converting agent that is structurally related to diuretics. It works by preventing the release of insulin from the pancreas and is commonly used in the treatment of hypoglycemia (low blood sugar). It offers some promise as an agent to promote hair growth but is still experimental for this purpose.

Because of multiple documented cases of hirsutism as a side effect of prolonged oral diazoxide therapy, Dr. Ken Hashimoto of Wayne State University became interested in topical diazoxide as a way to promote scalp hair growth. He used a stable 3 percent solution. In initial trials of 60 patients, about 25 percent had some visible mature hair growth, and the remainder had some intermediate hair growth. Only 1 patient had no response.

Although the experiments have not been concluded and there has been no follow-up after cessation of treatment, researchers think that, as with minoxidil, once the diazoxide treatments cease, hair will fall out. With the 3 percent solution of diazoxide being studied, no side effects have been noted to date.

VIPROSTOL

An antihypertensive drug, Viprostol is a synthetic prostaglandin E_2 (PGE) derivative that reduces blood pressure by direct dilation of the blood vessels. Like the other blood pressure medications used for hair loss, Viprostol appears to work by inducing the growth of hair when applied topically. At first, this drug was thought to be a step forward, because it is easily absorbed through the dermis, the second layer of the skin, which provides structural support, and shows marked penetration of the hair follicles. However, double-blind, placebo-controlled studies at Northwestern University and the University of North Carolina showed no effect by the drug on male pattern baldness; in fact, they indicated a significant decline in nonvellus hair growth in the target area over 24 weeks. And it has been determined that in contrast to the other blood vessel dilator, minoxidil, Viprostol has no hair-promoting effects in male pattern baldness. This drug has not been approved by the FDA.

∽
CYCLOSPORINE

An immunosuppressive agent used to prevent rejection of organ transplants, cyclosporine is also used to treat patients with severe psoriasis. In these individuals, cyclosporine was found to cause excessive hair growth on the body and scalp. This development prompted the experimental use of a topical cyclosporine solution in male pattern baldness. How or why the drug promotes hair growth is not known. It is thought that topical treatment with cyclosporine probably has a direct effect at the cellular level of the hair follicle and may change downy, fine hairs to mature hairs.

In two studies, applying 1 and 2 percent cyclosporine solutions twice daily to the scalp for four months, a small increase in hair count and decreased shedding were noted in approximately 20 percent of the patients in one of the studies. However, minimal changes were noted in the rest of the participants.

Cyclosporine should only be used topically. Further studies are seeking the most appropriate vehicle and concentration for a topical preparation. The oral form of cyclosporine is poorly absorbed topically and causes many side effects, including kidney dysfunction and lymphoma formation.

∽
RETINOIDS

Since their utilization in the treatment of acne began in 1982, retinoids have been shown to increase vellus and body hair. Consequently, it was felt that these vitamin A derivatives may stimulate the hair follicle.

This thesis gained further support after treti-noin (Retin-A) 0.025 percent solution was applied topically to the skin of vitamin A–deficient gerbils who had sparse fur development at four weeks. The gerbils developed normal coats of fur. Recently, pilot studies have been performed utilizing tretinoin (0.025 percent) in an alcoholic solution for treat-ment of male pattern baldness. Vellus hair has grown in a number of patients.

It is not fully understood why retinoids may be helpful in combating hair loss. They may be impor-tant in changing the status of regressing follicles, increasing the rate of hair growth, prolonging the active growth phase of the hair cycle, and playing a role in converting downy, almost invisible hairs to mature hairs.

— Another series of studies was performed on 36 patients using a combination of retinoids and min-oxidil. Moderate to good hair regrowth was noted in more than 50 percent of patients treated. It is thought that the combination works better than either of these drugs alone because the retinoid agents may act synergistically with minoxidil to pro-duce a more dense hair regrowth from regressing follicles. At present, larger controlled studies and better methods for assessing hair growth are neces-sary to support these early results.

There are side effects of retinoid treatment, however. Local irritation, peeling, and crusting may occur with the topical use of tretinoin. These effects appear to be dose related: the larger the dose the more extensive the irritation. This group of agents also may increase sun sensitivity in the skin.

The topical agents developed to date for the treatment of male pattern baldness have produced mixed results. On the negative side, no mechanical intervention has been shown to produce a full head of hair after a onetime use. All these agents probably require a lifetime commitment for even minimal results, all are expensive, and all have side effects that vary among individuals.

On the positive side, topical treatments do show promise. Their side effects are essentially controllable, the medications appear to be helpful in slowing the rate of hair loss, and this area of study seems to be opening the door to encouraging results.

It must be remembered that male pattern baldness is a cyclical phenomena. Hair is lost, hair stops growing, than it starts again. It is easy to assume incorrectly that a hair-growing product has actually stopped hair loss, if hair goes into a no-loss phase of the cycle while a particular product is being used. It is only with long-term follow-up that adequate evaluation of a given hair-growth-promoting agent can be made.

11

Surgical Procedures

According to ancient legends, it was the Japanese who first transplanted hair several centuries ago, when it was considered vital for a virginal young bride to have adequate pubic hair. Those not sufficiently supplied by nature were expected to have medical help. However, contemporary investigation into the possibilities of hair transplants actually began in 1954, when scientists observed that small, full-thickness scalp grafts taken from the hair-bearing posterior scalp continued to grow hair after having been moved to bald or thinning areas.

∽

TRANSPLANTS

The scientific name for what the average person calls a hair transplant is *donor dominance,* which simply means that hair follicles taken from the active areas of hair growth, which are genetically programmed to continue growing hair and never go completely bald, will grow hair regardless of where they are placed. Since the process began, over 2 million people of all races, sexes, and age groups have undergone successful medical hair transplants.

Of course, many improvements have been made in technique, instrumentation, design of hairlines, management of donor sites, and harvesting of grafts. Essentially, though, the same basic system of moving hair grafts from the active sites to the bald areas of an individual's head remains the foundation of hair transplants. The surgical procedure is relatively simple and straightforward, but many medical and practical nuances can contribute to good or bad results.

Patient Selection

Despite advances, not every individual is an appropriate candidate for the procedure.

To determine whether a patient is a viable subject for a hair transplant, the doctor performing the procedure will do three things:

1. Assess the donor area. That is, make sure the patient has sufficient active hair growth from which transplants can be made. Characteristics of the hair shaft, density of the hair, even the color and curl of the hair need to be taken into account.

2. Explain and detail the results that can be expected. Most male patients who seek advice on surgical hair restoration are between their twenties and forties; younger men rarely need the procedure, and older men have generally adjusted to the loss of their hair. However, it has been found that the younger the individual, the more unrealistic the expectations. The surgery most often results in a high hairline, which is acceptable to older patients but not to younger men. However, younger men with earlier stages of hair loss are better candidates because they usually have sufficient hair remaining to cover transplant sites while they are healing and before hair regrowth.

3. Make sure the candidate is committed to the procedure. Depending on the extent of hair loss and amount of hair to be transplanted, an individual may need to return for multiple sessions for as long as one to two years.

Three areas of consideration make a patient a more or less appropriate candidate for a hair transplant.

PHYSICAL STATE OF THE HAIR The less hair that needs to be transplanted, the easier and less expensive the procedure will be. With patients whose hair loss is minimal, it is possible and relatively simple to keep a high hairline. On individuals who have lost a great deal of hair, it is more difficult to create full maximum-density replacement.

Thin-caliber hair is more difficult to transplant than thick-caliber hair because it doesn't provide the cross-sectional density to cover as much of the bald scalp. Consequently, it takes more hair per square inch to give the appearance of full hair. Also, thin-caliber hair does not provide the lift of a thick hair shaft, which contributes to a full look. It is difficult to improve the quality of an individual's hair, but cosmetic conditioners may help by precipitating protein into the hair shaft, thus giving the hair a fuller appearance.

Although dark hair usually looks the thickest and most full, salt-and-pepper or blond are the preferred colors for hair transplants because they blend into the surrounding hair better. However, darker hair that doesn't look right after a transplant can be colored to blend in with the hair color around it.

Curly or wavy hair provides the best coverage because it bends into itself, making the hair appear fuller. The person who has transplanted straight hair can, however, have a professional permanent, which will give the hair a thicker appearance. Hair can be cut and permed as soon as it grows to sufficient length. Transplanted hair grows at the same rate as nontransplanted hair, that is, 1½ to 2 inches every three months (0.37 mm a day).

GENDER   It is more difficult to achieve acceptable hair transplant results on women than on men for three reasons:

1. Women tend to be less satisfied with the final results of hair transplants.
2. Many women who seek a hair transplant have diffuse hair loss, which affects not only the male pattern area of the head but also the sides and back of the scalp. Consequently, they have limited areas of high-density hair from which to take donor plugs.
3. Even when a woman's hair loss is confined

to the male pattern areas, the progression of loss may continue in the donor sites, causing a decrease in the number of mature hairs in the transplanted grafts.

HEALTH STATES Although hair transplants have been performed on patients in their eighties and nineties, and virtually anyone in good basic health can be considered for the procedure, there are some medical conditions that rule out a hair transplant, need to be taken into consideration, or must be cured before the transplant can proceed.

Diabetics who require insulin should be treated with care, as should hypertensive individuals. Medical control of these conditions should be achieved before a hair transplant so as not to exacerbate them. Patients on beta-blocker therapy should be tapered off the drugs before having a hair transplant because epinephrine is often employed as one of the anesthetic agents in the procedure.

Inflammatory skin disease, such as psoriasis and seborrheic dermatitis, need to be successfully treated before surgery. Active infections, such as herpes simplex and hepatitis, should also be cured before transplants begin. Active herpes simplex may spread if it is present at the time of surgery.

Pretransplant Planning

Before undergoing a hair transplant, the patient should expect the doctor to explain six items in detail:

1. The number of grafts and any other surgical procedures, such as removal of parts of a balding scalp (scalp reductions), that the patient will require. If the patient is a candidate for scalp reduction surgery, donor hair sites can be conserved and the number of hair transplant grafts necessary to cover the balding area decreased.

2. The approximate cost. Hair transplantation is a cosmetic procedure, so payment is usually required at the time of the visit. The cost per graft varies from $20 to $50 (50 to 125 grafts are performed at a time). Scalp reduction procedures cost from $2,000 to $5,000, depending on the degree of scalp removed and the experience and expertise of the surgeon. The total cost of the transplant depends on the number of scalp transplants and scalp reduction procedures utilized and ranges from $2,000 to $15,000. Up to 350 grafts may be required for a diffusely balding scalp.

3. The time involved in the transplant session and the entire process.

4. The number of transplants required; in other words, the number of grafts needed for coverage of balding areas and the number of transplant sessions necessary. Three to four hundred grafts transplanted in three to five sessions is usual.

5. The sequence of transplants; in other words, what areas will be done first.

6. The time before final results can be seen and the expected outcome of the procedure.

The plan of treatment can vary based on the degree of hair loss to be replaced, the cosmetic need to cover the healing but not yet growing grafts, whether scalp reduction will be done, how often the procedure will be performed, and the transplant sequence.

When considering a hair transplant surgeon, ask to see pre- and postoperative photographs. You may also request the telephone numbers of one or two patients who have had transplants in order to gain some personal insight into the procedure.

The Plug Procedure

On the morning of the hair transplant, patients are instructed to cleanse their hair with an antiseptic shampoo.

At the doctor's office, a painkiller is given. Relaxing sedatives, such as Valium, may be used as well as nitrous oxide to decrease the patient's apprehension and lower the pain threshold. Next, the donor and the balding areas are cleansed with an antiseptic solution and a local anesthesia, lidocaine compounded with epinephrine, is administered.

A power punch, an electrically driven device, is used to take the donor grafts (called *plugs*) from back of fringe areas of the scalp, and a hand or power punch is employed to prepare the balding areas for the donor grafts. A full plug is round, 2 to 4 millimeters in diameter, and may be divided into four wedge-shaped sections called *miniplugs*, which are used with full plugs for a more natural appearance. After the local anesthesia is administered, there is little pain during the procedure. The donor site is chosen so that there will be minimal scarring; it is usually the back or side of the scalp, where it is concealed by the surrounding hair. The grafts are trimmed of some fat, then placed into the recipient sites. There is little blood loss. In most procedures,

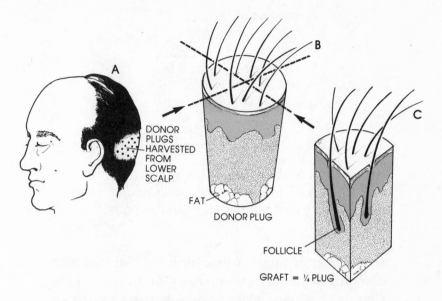

FIGURE **11-1.** *Hair Plug Containing Follicle and Hair. A 4.75-millimeter round plug of tissue is harvested from a hair-growing area of the scalp with a punch. It is then divided into four wedge-shaped sections with a scalpel. Some fat is usually scraped away before it is transplanted.*

there is an average of 15 to 20 growing hairs in each full plug graft.

Transplant sessions usually last from one to two hours. A bandage is applied after the procedure and is usually removed at the physician's office the following morning. There may be mild to moderate pain the first night after the procedure. However, this can easily be controlled with pain medication.

Although a doctor may alter the plan as it goes along, three to five sessions are usually planned at first. The frontal hairline is established in the first ses-

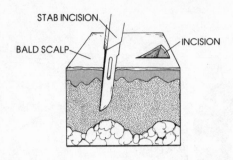

FIGURE **11-2.** *Stab Incision. Site preparation consists of a single stab incision made with scalpel blade to create a recipient bed for each quarter graft.*

sion. The graft plugs are placed with slightly less than one-plug diameter between rows. At the second session, plugs are placed between the previous implants. If the first plugs are correctly placed, the second series will fit closely between them. At sessions three and four, the spaces between the rows are filled in. And the procedure continues in this fashion.

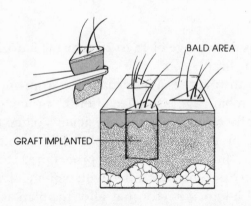

FIGURE **11-3.** *Transplant Procedure. Jeweler's forceps insert a quarter graft into a prepared stab incision.*

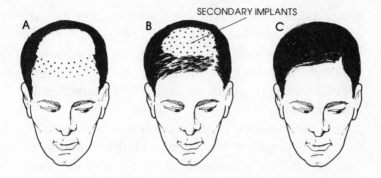

FIGURE **11-4.** *Hair Transplant. (A) Donor plugs harvested from lower scalp and hairline established; (B) hair growth in front with later transplants behind; (C) full growth of new hair.*

Spaces are left between grafts and multiple procedures are required in order to allow the grafts to receive adequate nutrient blood supply. After 8 to 12 weeks, the blood supply has been established and new grafts can be added. With new suturing techniques, the scalp at the donor sites is cosmetically closed, and it is ultimately covered by the surrounding hair. When the whole procedure is finished, no balding sites remain in the donor areas.

Other Transplant Procedures

Along with the basic plug transplant procedure, four variations are also used.

MICRO AND MINI GRAFTING These procedures employ one to three (micro) and three to five hair-bearing grafts (mini) to fill in around and between larger grafts. Micro and mini grafting produce a more nat-ural-looking hairline and crown. These small, angu-lated grafts provide a finer, feathered appearance, counteracting the cornstalk, irregular shape of the normal hair transplant, which is often cosmetically unacceptable.

These grafts can also be employed to grow hair on scars secondary to trauma, infection, inflamma-tory disease, or radiation, or to reconstruct eye-brows.

BLEND GRAFTING   This procedure entails the use of grafts of various sizes placed at special angles within the newly created hairline to achieve a completely natural look approaching that of the patient's origi-nal hairline.

STRIP GRAFTING   This process involves taking whole strips of hair from the donor area to the recipient sites. It is sometimes attempted to avoid the long, painstaking single-plug procedure. However, strip grafting has not produced the same density of growth as individual grafts and often causes slightly more scarring of the scalp.

INCISIONAL SLIT GRAFTING   This method uses micro and mini grafts to help develop a feathering zone hairline and minimize the cobblestone effect of the transplant plugs alone.

The Outcome

Most patients are able to resume their usual activi-ties and return to work in a day or two following a

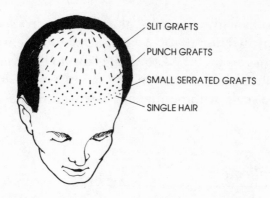

SLIT GRAFTS

PUNCH GRAFTS

SMALL SERRATED GRAFTS

SINGLE HAIR

FIGURE **11-5.** *Transplants on a Nearly Bald Man. Note full plug grafts, slit grafts, and micro and mini grafts. Note single-hair grafts along the hairline to create a natural appearance.*

hair transplant. Possible discomfort the first postoperative night is treated with a mild pain-relieving drug.

Some transplant surgeons suture the recipient grafts. However, this is unnecessary because the grafts tend to settle into place and are incorporated into the recipient tissue bed in 48 to 72 hours. When sutures are placed in the donor site, the stitches are removed in 7 to 10 days.

As the scalp heals, crusts form over the recipient sites; they tend to fall off spontaneously within two weeks, but they can be removed mechanically by the physician. With the latest techniques, the donor site shows virtually no sign of hair removal.

Donor grafts are placed in the balding areas at an angle that duplicates the hair's natural growth pattern, producing a thick, natural-looking head of hair similar to what the patient had originally. However, because the hair goes into a resting phase after the transplant procedure, the patient won't see new hair growth for 10 to 12 weeks. Once the active hair cycle is reestablished, the hair grows at the same rate as natural hair (½ to ¾ inch a month), covering the entire scalp with permanent hair within one to two years.

Complications

Despite the advances in hair transplants, there may be complications:

Bleeding can usually be controlled with pressure bandaging and immobilization, as well as through the avoidance of blood-thinning medications that interfere with clotting, such as aspirin, before the procedure. Although the scalp is a remarkably vascular part of the body, it is amazing how little bleeding there is with expert technique and appropriate bandaging.

Scarring can occur where a large width of skin has been removed and closed under tension. However, because of the vascular nature of the scalp, scarring tends to be minimal and can usually be covered by surrounding hair.

Cobblestoning (irregular bumps on the head) is a rare problem. If it occurs, it can be touched up with light electrosurgical planing.

Frontal swelling (edema) may occur a couple of days following the hair transplant, particularly after the first session. However, this condition resolves quickly on its own.

Vascular abnormalities are extremely rare. However, it is possible for small blood vessels to deflate or for small vessels between the artery and vein to break. These conditions can be easily treated by tying off the blood vessels or injecting steroids into the scalp.

Inflammatory skin problems, such as seborrheic dermatitis or psoriasis, occasionally occur or may flare up following a hair transplant. They can be treated by standard measures.

Altered sensation, such as numbness or tingling above the donor site, is not uncommon. This condition usually resolves within three to four months. It is the result of the healing of tissues with associated regeneration of nerves after the surgical procedure.

Shedding can occur after the surgery because the transplanted hairs go into a resting phase. The stubble comes out when the scabs fall off and the hair begins to grow naturally. However, the trauma of surgery can affect both the donor and recipient areas, causing all the surrounding hairs to go into a resting phase. Adjacent hair plugs may also be affected each time new plugs are inserted. The shedding that follows can be both emotionally and cosmetically upsetting. However, the condition usually corrects itself in 9 to 12 months.

Inadequate growth of the transplanted hair can be caused by a number of factors:

- Strenuous exercise too soon after surgery
- The physician's cutting and grafting at angles that are not parallel to the hair shafts, causing destruction of the follicles under the hair that is transplanted
- The use of dull instruments, which can twist the graft, resulting in poor growth

- Excessive drying of the grafts during the procedure
- Crushing of the grafts with forceps during their insertion, damaging the hair follicles
- Too many grafts placed in too small an area, compromising the blood supply
- Grafts that are too large for the recipient site
- Not enough time allowed between transplant sessions for the nutrient blood supply to be established
- Sparse donor areas
- Cutting of the hair follicles while thinning the fat from the base of the graft. Many, though not all, hair transplant surgeons trim the fat off grafts before implanting them. Although those who perform this step claim that the trimmed grafts take better, dissenting surgeons say that trimming the grafts often damages the hair follicle. Certainly, too vigorous thinning of the fat from the graft will result in damage to some or all of the hair follicles.

The patient should expect virtually 100 percent success of donor grafts. Each graft contains an average of 12 to 15 hairs. The problems that arise from hair transplant surgery can almost always be treated and controlled. The viability of the transplanted hair can be directly linked to the expertise and technique of the surgeon.

SCALP REDUCTION

Scalp reduction, the surgical removal of balding areas of scalp, was initially discussed in 1978 by

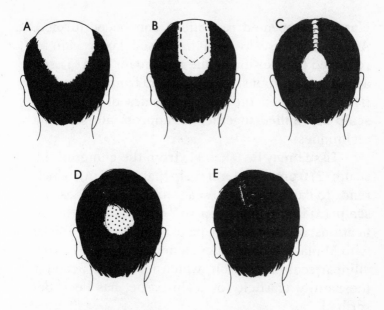

FIGURE **11-6.** *Scalp Reduction. Figures A (before treatment) through E (after treatment) show how several scalp reduction procedures, the last with the addition of punch grafting to cover the remaining bald spot (D), can result in a full head of hair.*

researchers at the International Hair Transplant Symposium in Lucerne, Switzerland. This procedure, when used in conjunction with a hair transplant, can dramatically improve cosmetic results because it cuts down the area of balding scalp without reducing any of the available donor areas.

Procedure

A local anesthesia is applied to the area, and the sections to be excised are outlined (an average of 12 to 16 inches is removed per procedure) from the middle or side of the scalp. Depending on the scalp's elasticity, repeated reductions can be performed. Areas of the scalp with increased laxity can be removed by excision of the redundant area. Tissue around the cutout sites is loosened from its connective tissue, then the opposing sides of remaining scalp are pulled together by appropriate suturing techniques.

Tissue may be taken (1) from the center of the scalp; (2) from the lateral scalp (paramedian), which tends to camouflage the scar along the hair-bearing scalp; (3) in the shape of a Y (Y-plasty) and its modifications; or (4) in the shape of a modified M (ellipse with M-plasty). In addition, a new technique of curvilinear scalp reduction, which takes into account the natural elasticity of scalp tissue, has been described.

In some cases, scalp expanders, balloons that inflate the scalp, can be inserted either before or during the scalp reduction procedure. The expander stretches the scalp, allowing the surgeon to remove as much as 50 percent more skin at a session.

Most patients prefer to have the expander inserted at the time of the surgery rather than earlier. Even though more skin can be removed if the balloon is placed in a separate, earlier procedure, surgical insertion of the expander requires that the area be allowed to heal before the scalp reduction is commenced, so the patient can be walking around with a bulging deformity of the scalp for up to six weeks.

The Outcome

The scalp reduction procedure is most often utilized on patients who have loose, redundant scalp. It is sometimes done alone, particularly to cover scars, but most often it is done in conjunction with transplants. It has the following advantages for transplant patients:

1. It minimizes the number of grafts necessary to cover a balding area.
2. It makes transplants possible in some patients with too few donor areas.
3. It allows complete correction in some patients with only crown or central loss of hair.
4. It can vary or change the position of the part and help correct previous poorly done transplants.

Complications

Possible complications and problems with scalp reduction include the following:

1. Pain for the first 24 hours. This is treatable with pain medication.
2. Infection.
3. Stretchback. Sometimes the tissue re-expands. This occurs in 10 to 50 percent of scalp reduction procedures. However, more sophisticated techniques are helping to minimize this complication.
4. Scarring. This can be minimized with appropriate planning, which places transplanted hair to cover the scars.
5. Distortion of the bald area as a result of bad surgical technique.

6. Decreased density of the donor hair at the sides of the head. This problem is the result of poor surgical work.

The cost of scalp reduction is between $2,000 and $5,000.

❧

SCALP FLAPS

Because of complications associated with this procedure, scalp flaps remain controversial. Scalp flap surgery is the process of moving a piece of hair-bearing scalp into a bald area. There are two major types of flaps: Juri flap and TPO (temporo-parietal-occipital) flap. The Juri flap is used for taking sections from the sides of the head and moving them toward the front. The TPO flap is moved from the back and sides of the head onto the front or top.

Patient Selection

The key to successful scalp flap surgery is patient selection. It is too often possible for a scalp flap to look unreal. The most appropriate patient for this procedure has only frontal baldness with dark, coarse hairs behind. Then the scalp flap will cover the bald area and blend well into the surrounding hair. However, if the patient has frontal baldness and thinning hair behind, a scalp flap will resemble an island of hair. Sometimes micro or mini transplants in front of a frontal scalp flap help disguise the sharp outlines of the hair.

The Procedure

For scalp flap surgery, a local anesthesia (lidocaine with epinephrine) is employed. The flap is outlined, and its vascular nutrient supply located. The flap is cut out, then sutured into a prepared recipient site, and the head is fully bandaged. Steroids, antibiotics, and painkillers are given after the surgery.

The patient recieves a second, modifying procedure usually six weeks after the initial operation and scalp reduction to remove bald scalp between flaps or between a flap and a balding area. In addition, plug hair transplants may be carried out in sites of baldness not covered by the flap.

Advantages

There are several advantages to scalp flaps:

- The results are immediate. By contrast, cosmetic results from transplants are delayed a minimum of six months and can take years.
- The transposed hair is thicker than the hair that can be transplanted.
- On heads that have dense, natural hairlines behind the flap, the frontal dense hairline cannot be accomplished with any other technique.
- A single flap in a bald crown covers with

excellent density and leaves the hair easier to style and manage than it is immediately following scalp reductions.

Complications

However, there are also problems with scalp flaps, and it is vital that the patient be aware of both the cosmetic and medical risks associated with this procedure. There is usually a six- to seven-week convalescence period following surgery. Careful postoperative monitoring of vital signs, bleeding, and swelling is required. Also, tissue death *(necrosis)*, caused when a flap fails to take, can lead to ulceration and scarring of the scalp. This condition is particularly risky for patients who smoke, have diabetes, or have collagen vascular diseases such as lupus erythematosus. Another complication is the possibility of scarring in the donor area. This scarring can spread with associated traumatic or patchy baldness. The size and extent of the flap can be discouraging, as can be the unnaturalness of the resulting hair pattern. Several scalp reductions are usually necessary to eliminate remaining baldness.

At present, hair transplants provide the one means by which men with balding areas on the top of their heads can achieve a full head of hair. But it must be stressed that any surgical hair-replacement procedure must be undertaken only after the patient has investigated his case and the procedure thoroughly. And, again, the expertise of the surgeon can make the procedure either rewarding or disastrous.

12

Hair Prosthetics

WIGS

A wig is a hairpiece designed to cover either a portion of the head or the entire head. Despite the ongoing sly references and jokes that hairpieces provoke, wigs have been around since ancient times. The Egyptians shaved and plucked their hair, then put on wigs. This procedure was for religious observances, for cleanliness, and, in that warm country, to keep the wearer cool. The length of a wig depended on the wealth of the wearer. The Romans equipped their statues with removable marble wigs, which were often changed so that the honored could keep up with the latest hairstyles.

In the sixteenth century men and women of virtually every level of society around the world had wigs in elaborate styles that took months to create and were often worn until they disintegrated. Because cleanliness was not a major consideration during this time, it was not unusual for vermin and other small creatures to make their homes in the larger wigs.

In America, wigs have slipped into and out of vogue. Considered frivolous by many early American colonists, wigs were nevertheless worn by some of the founders of our country. Today over 2 million American men and women wear hairpieces, paying between $325 and $2,000 for women's wigs and $1,000 to $3,500 for men's. This results in an outlay of approximately $350 million annually.

The products of the wig industry are made of one of three materials:

Human hair wigs are the most expensive. The hair for these hairpieces has never been colored, bleached, or permed. The color of these wigs reacts to the sun.

Animal hair wigs can be made from the hair of goats, horses, monkeys, dogs, or yaks. These are most often used for white or silver wigs.

Synthetic wigs are made of nylon or other man-made materials. These are the cheapest wigs and can be purchased for under $50. The best of these wigs currently come from France, where the latest synthetic wigs are water resistant, hold styles well, and can look like real hair.

The best and most expensive wigs are hand tied, which makes them both fragile and real looking because hairs are knotted to the cap individually, much the way human hair grows.

Machine-made wigs are sewn in spirals around the netting or wig cap. These wigs are usually firmer than the hand tied and will hold their shape longer, but they don't have the loose, natural look of a hand-tied wig.

A good combination is a machine-sewn wig that is hand finished, which gives a natural hairline.

The caps themselves can be made from cotton, silk, or nylon (which will shrink). Lighter fabrics keep the head cool; heavier fabrics hold their shape better.

If worn regularly, however, a wig can cause the glands in the scalp to produce more oil than usual. Moreover, often the scalp sweats under a hairpiece. If a wig is worn on a long-term basis, a person's own hair can become unkempt and oily, which may lead to inflammation of the hair follicles. And wearing a wig may exacerbate dandruff in individuals who have this problem as a consequence of the rise in the temperature of the scalp.

A company in California has recently introduced a wig designed for women suffering from the side effects of chemotherapy or alopecia areata. Created to look and feel completely natural, the hairpiece can be shampooed, permed, colored, and styled. It features a breathable mesh cap, sculpted to follow the natural hairline. Its most novel feature is that it allows the scalp to breathe.

∽

HAIR WEAVING

Hair weaving is accomplished by attaching a piece of false hair to an individual's own hair with nylon thread. The false hair used for this procedure can be human or synthetic. It is attached as close as possible to the scalp, usually in a ready-made matching color. Then the hair is cut, styled, and blended with the natural hair. This process takes about two hours to complete. Woven hair will loosen over time, growing away from the scalp, and have to be adjusted.

Cleanliness is a problem, however, because woven hair cannot be washed as frequently and vigorously as normal hair. It is also impossible to change the style without removing the weaves, and the hair must be styled down on the forehead to cover the front hairline.

IMPLANTS

This is partially a medical procedure and partially a cosmetic one. There are several types of implants. Some provide anchoring for a full wig. Others provide a method of attaching false hair directly to the scalp.

If the full wig method is to be used, a plaster of paris mold of the patient's head is made and false hair, the same color and texture as the patient's, is custom-made into a wig that fits the mold. The manufacture of such a wig usually takes between 10 and 21 days.

In the actual implant procedure, the patient's scalp is injected with a local anesthetic. Suture material is implanted into the fatty tissue of the scalp, and the uncut hair implant (called a *unit*) is attached to the sutures.

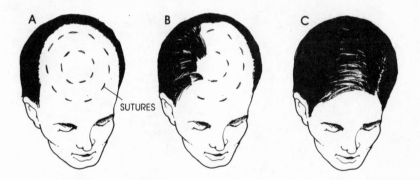

FIGURE **12-1.** *Cosmetic Suture. Surgical stitches are implanted all over the bald area. Then strands of artificial hair are attached to the stitches, resulting in the appearance of a full head of hair.*

The hair is then cut and styled as the patient chooses. After the implant is secured and styled, the patient's own hair is pulled up through the implant net and blended into the new hair.

A variation of this procedure dispenses with the wig and places multiple sutures at intervals on the bare scalp. False hair is drawn through the sutures and mingled with natural hair.

The drawbacks to implants are similar to the general problems of wearing a wig except they are more severe. The sweating, oiliness, and cleanliness difficulties can all be present. Implants have fallen out of favor because of problems with severe infections and scarring as well as foreign-body reactions, which can be life-threatening. This method of hair replacement should be avoided.

PART FOUR

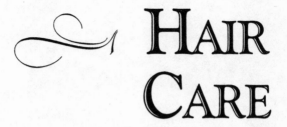

HAIR CARE

13

Hair Cosmetics

There is no question that hair plays an integral and important part in virtually every individual's self-image and the way he or she is looked upon by society. To this end, cosmetic companies, hair salons, hair-loss centers, and a wide range of other inventive individuals try to persuade people to use specific products or methods to improve hair condition. Hair is in many ways like a fine fabric. It needs to be washed with the proper soap, carefully dried, and shaped to retain its maximum appearance—just like an expensive wool sweater.

∾
SHAMPOOS

Today the average American shampoos his or her hair two to seven times a week. And, because

144 · HAIR CARE

such frequent washing is a relatively new phenomenon, the cosmetics industry has moved toward products that can be used this frequently. The basic
purpose of a hair shampoo is to remove sebum residue and foreign materials (dirt, hair spray, gels,
mousses, and so on) from the hair and to cleanse the
hair and scalp.

The choice of shampoo depends on type of hair,
the presence or absence of sun damage, whether the
individual is also using permanent-wave solutions or
hair-coloring products, and, of course, personal
preference.

Although shampoos can vary somewhat, the
major components of most are water, detergent, and
fatty material. The pH levels of shampoos can also
vary, but for normal hair a pH range of 7.5 to 8.5 is
suggested. Shampoo with a higher pH level will
clean hair more thoroughly but can be too harsh for
even normal hair. For hair that has been bleached,
dyed, or chemically straightened, a shampoo with a
lower pH is recommended.

Soap Shampoos

These products are made of sodium hydroxide or
potassium hydroxide (alkali) combined with oils
(such as olive, coconut, or vegetable) or animal fats
(such as tallow or lanolin). They are available as gels,
granules, liquids, or bars.

Soap shampoos effectively remove dirt and
grease from the hair and scalp. But they can create a
scum when combined with hard water.

Detergent Shampoos

These are essentially oils treated with wetting agents (to enhance the product's ability to lather). The main ingredient in detergent shampoos is sulfonated oil. Detergent shampoos are available as powders, gels, creams, or liquids.

Because detergent shampoos are made from synthetic petroleum products, they have one advantage over soap shampoos: They do not produce hard-water scum. Their principal surfactants (the surface-active agents that give these products their cleaning and foaming power) come from anionic (negatively charged) substances, such as alkyl-sulfates, made from alcohols obtained from the fatty acids of coconut and palm kernel oil. Secondary surfactants add to the foaming power of detergent shampoos as well as improve and condition the hair.

Dry Shampoos

These products are made of orrisroot, talc, chalk, and starch and are used without water or lathering. They contain emulsifying agents that dissolve and absorb oils and dirt from the hair shaft.

SHAMPOO ADDITIVES

In addition to basic ingredients that cause shampoos to cleanse and foam, shampoos can contain a number of additives designed for specific purposes.

Germicides (antibacterial agents) are added to shampoos to create medicated preparations designed for the treatment of seborrheic dermatitis or other scalp disorders. They may include tar, which functions as an anti-inflammatory agent; sulfur, selenium disulfide, or zinc pyrithione, which acts as an antibacterial and antifungal agent; or salicylic acid, which aids in scalp scale removal.

Conditioners are usually added to shampoos specifically meant for use on chemically treated hair. They can be detergent based, such as stearalkonium chloride or polyvinyl pyrrolidone (**PVP**), or contain nondetergent natural polymers; fatty materials (lanolin); or other natural products, such as herbs, peptides, or substances derived from eggs.

Sequestrants are texturizers added to treat damaged hair.

Thickeners impart a rich feel to the shampoo.

Opacifiers are designed to impart a specific appearance to the hair, for instance, highlights.

Shampoos can also contain color (for brightening hair), perfumes, preservatives, heavy detergents (for oily hair), or amphoteric detergents (gentle detergents such as are found in baby shampoos).

∽

CONDITIONERS

Hair that is totally devoid of sebum is subject to static electricity, harsh to the touch, and dull in appearance. This condition can result from the use or overuse of heavy detergent shampoos.

Because the more thorough shampoos cause sebum to be removed from the hair shaft and can damage the cuticle of the hair, conditioners were invented to rectify these problems. It is, in some respects, a catch-22 situation. The cosmetic companies recognized (or helped create) the public's interest in very clean hair. Having manufactured the shampoos to accomplish this purpose, they then began providing conditioners to repair the damage resulting from use of aggressive shampoos. Of course, if a person doesn't use heavy detergent shampoos, then his or her hair will be less likely to need a conditioner.

Conditioners are primarily designed to control dry, flyaway hair; restore manageability, softness, and shine to the hair; impart a thicker feel to the hair shaft; and coat and give body to damaged hair.

There are three basic categories of conditioning agents:

1. Cationic (positively charged) detergent conditioners. These conditioners contain quaternary ammonium compounds and work by depositing a positively charged film on a negatively charged damaged hair shaft. In other words, neutralizing the negative charge surrounding damaged or chemically processed (dyed) hair will soothe the hair cuticle and restore manageability, softness, and shine to the hair.
2. Film-forming conditioners. Based on polymers that coat the hair shaft, reducing static

electricity, these conditioners also fill in surface cuticle defects.

3. Protein-based conditioners. These are currently very popular because of their ability to penetrate the hair shaft and recondition damaged hair.

Protein is lost from hair during excessive hair grooming (brushing) or as a result of chemical processing. The effect of a protein conditioner is most likely temporary, because much of the residual protein is removed by the next shampooing.

The protein used in protein-based conditioners comes from a variety of sources. However, the source of protein is not nearly as important as the way the protein is treated and produced. In order to be truly effective, the protein in a conditioner must be hydrolyzed into fragments actually small enough to penetrate the hair shaft.

Hair conditioners include four types:

1. Instant conditioners are liquid. They are applied to the hair following shampooing, left on for a few minutes, then rinsed out.
2. Liquid conditioners are left in place on the hair. They are often recognizable as blow-drying lotions, hair thickeners, or hair glazes.
3. Deep conditioners are left on freshly shampooed hair for 20 to 30 minutes, with or without the application of infrared heat or a heat cap. (Heat encourages the product to penetrate the hair shaft by increasing swelling of the hair cuticle.)
4. Extra-deep conditioners are used only

every week or two. These products consist of hydrolyzed animal protein applied with a hot pack that opens the cuticle so that the keratin or collagen can penetrate the hair shaft and be deposited in the cortex of the hair. This procedure is most appropriate for hair that is badly damaged. It is also used before color or wave treatments, because it encourages the new color or perm to take evenly by improving the hair's porosity.

RINSES

A rinse is ostensibly intended to untangle hair. Because the major aim of a rinse is to remove the surface film of soap, allowing the hair to be combed easily, the traditional agents—vinegar (for dark hair) and lemon (for light hair), which through their acidity counteract the alkaline nature of soap—are still popular as natural rinses.

Beeswax or paraffin (such as in balsam conditioners) are also rinse agents, adding a slippery film to the hair to ease a comb's passage through it.

PERMANENT WAVING

Human hair has three types of wave patterns: straight, wavy, and kinky. Since the time of Cleopatra humans have been trying to change the type they inherited. In 1905 Charles Nessler invented the heat permanent-waving machine. This innovation was followed in the 1930s by the cold-wave process, using the alkaline ammonium thioglycolate. And in 1970 the acid-based glycerol monothioglycolate perm was invented. All three methods act by breaking the disulfide bonds in the hair, then restoring the bonds once the hair has been placed in its new form.

Acid permanent waves employ a waving lotion with a pH of 7.0 to 8.8 that may consist of thioglycolic acid buffered with ammonium bicarbonate or the glycerol ester of thioglycolic acid, glycerol mono-thioglycolate (GMTG). These perms require either heat applied by a hair dryer or the inherent heat of the scalp, which can be trapped by placing a plastic bag over the hair. Acid permanents usually produce a soft, loose curl and are generally recommended for damaged or chemically treated hair. However, hair stylists often incur contact dermatitis from acid solutions; consequently, it is recommended that gloves be worn by the person applying the treatment.

Alkaline permanents employ a pH between 9 and 10. They do not require heat and take effect more quickly than acid permanent waves. The result of this treatment is usually a tight, long-lasting curl. But the hair may suffer considerable damage, resulting in frizziness or harsh appearance.

Sulfite permanents are the most common types of home treatments. These products usually are odor free, are only moderately damaging to the hair shaft, and normally produce soft, short-lived curls.

Steps

The first step in giving a permanent is to shampoo the hair. This brings water into the hydrogen bonds in the hair shaft, resulting in increased flexibility.

Next the hair is sectioned into 30 to 50 areas, depending on hair length and thickness, and wrapped on mandrels. The size of the mandrels determines the size of the curl; large mandrels yield larger curls, small mandrels yield smaller curls. The tension applied to the hair as it is wrapped can also affect the size of the curl. For example, if the hair is pulled firmly around the mandrel, the curl will be tighter than if the hair is wrapped loosely.

Following the wrapping process, the hair is thoroughly saturated with a waving lotion (acid, alkaline, or sulfite), which remains in place for 5 to 20 minutes. Hair that has never had a permanent or any prior chemical treatments is more resistant to the process and will likely require a longer time in the solution.

Once the waving lotion is removed, a neutralizing solution containing hydrogen peroxide combined with other chemicals is applied to re-form the disulfide bonds in the hair's new position. How long the permanent lasts depends on the type of lotion used and how it is applied.

∽

HAIR STRAIGHTENERS

Hair can be straightened or relaxed by three methods.

MECHANICAL STRAIGHTENING Pomades containing a combination of heavy vegetable and mineral oils and petrolatum are used. They have limited value in actually straightening the hair, but the weight of the pomade causes the hair to flatten out and lie closer to the scalp, giving the appearance of straightness. In some individuals, grease occlusion resulting from the use of these products may produce secondary acne–type reactions.

HEAT STRAIGHTENING   Hot combing uses a metal comb that is heated to between 200° and 500°F, then drawn through the hair. This process causes the reformable bonds of the hair to break, thus allowing the hair to be pulled straight. In hair pressing the hair is ironed between metal plates, thus breaking the reformable bonds and straightening the hair. Neither of these procedures is permanent. Heat straightening is immediately reversible if the hair gets wet from perspiration, humidity, shampooing, and so on.

Pressing oil increases the heat transfer to the hair and repels moisture. Consequently, the application of a pressing oil to the hair before hot combing can lengthen the time before regression. However, this product can also contribute to irreversible inflammation of the hair follicles and subsequent scarring alopecia (hot comb alopecia).

CHEMICAL STRAIGHTENING   This procedure is similar to permanent waving, except that, instead of being wrapped around mandrels, the hair shafts are combed straight following applications of a disulfide bond–breaking preparation. The chemical products for straightening hair are identical to permanent-wave solutions, except that they are formulated as thick creams rather than lotions to add weight, thus aiding in holding the hair straight.

Hair straighteners are made of thioglycolate or lye-based creams. Because of the lye (and the possible addition of up to a 3 percent sodium hydroxide in some of these products), hair-straightening preparations can produce burns on the scalp or even blindness if allowed to drip into the eye. Newer, safer products replace the lye with quanidine hydroxide or lithium hydroxide. All these products can cause local irritation or allergic reactions.

∽

STYLING PREPARATIONS

A wide variety of styling preparations are available. Despite their many names and promotional titles, they can be basically classified as hair sprays, gels, or styling lotions.

Hair sprays are designed to help the hair stay in place, stiffening the hair so that it will retain a particular shape, curl, or orientation, either natural or imposed.

The original hair sprays containing natural resins (shellacs) are no longer used because of the difficulty in removing them from the hair. Today hair sprays contain copolymers such as PVP in an aerosol delivery system and are generally applied after styling. Other ingredients in most modern hair sprays include plasticizers, humectants (which help the hair retain moisture), solvents, conditioners, fragrance, and vinyl acetate (which improves hold under moist conditions, such as high humidity or perspiration). The concentration of copolymers in the spray determines the amount of hold.

Gels contain the same PVP and vinyl acetate copolymers as hair sprays. Application directly to the hair shaft by the delivery system of a gel provides greater hold than is possible with a hair spray because the amount of product deposited is increased. As with sprays, the amount of hold depends on the concentration of copolymers. Extremely high-hold gel products that lock the hair in place may contain methacrylate copolymers.

Styling lotions or hair-setting lotions are usually applied to towel-dried or dry hair before styling. Before the development of electric blow dryers, curlers, curling irons, and crimping irons, hairstyling was commonly done by shaping the hair on wire or plastic rollers, wrapping it with cloth, or shaping it with metal or plastic hair clips. At that time a styling lotion was applied to the slightly moist hair to increase the hold of the curl.

This method is rarely used today because of the invention of modern appliances; however, styling lotions are still popular because they can provide hold and firmness.

It should be noted that just as a gel is the same as a spray in a different form, a *mousse* is essentially a foaming version of the basic styling lotion. The inclusion of foam decreases the amount of hold provided. However, because the foam is easier to manipulate, it can be applied to hair after it has been dried, to the ends of the hair after they have been set, and to particular areas of the hair to increase hold.

∽

HAIR-COLORING PRODUCTS

Hair-coloring procedure and products have been around for centuries. The ancient Egyptians used henna packs to produce an orange-red coloration; Roman women, enamored of northern European slaves' blond hair, used lye and exposure to the sun to lighten their locks. These methods, as primitive as they may seem to us, were the basis of all hair coloring until the nineteenth century, when researchers began to develop modern hair-coloring procedures.

Today there is a wide range of processes capable of altering hair color. But basically all fall into one of five categories: temporary, gradual, natural, semipermanent, or permanent.

Temporary Colorants (Rinses)

The development of synthetic textile dyes led to their reformulation as temporary hair colorants or rinses. Basically, rinses are blends of four dyes, which produce a variety of shades according to how much of each goes into the mixture. Rinses are primarily used to modify gray hair. However, they are also employed by blonds for party colors, used to impart highlights to dull hair, and tried by individuals afraid to dye their hair permanently but wanting to experience a change of color. The major advantage of a temporary hair colorant is that it washes out easily with shampoo and rarely, if ever, causes any allergic reaction.

Gradual Colorants

During the nineteenth century, it was discovered that colorless solutions of lead salts applied daily to the hair would slowly build up a yellow-brown coloration. This development resulted in the marketing of color restorers, which can be more accurately described as gradual hair colorants. Modern gradual hair colorants are created from metallic salts, such as lead acetate and silver nitrate; the best-known product is made from an aqueous solution of lead acetate and glycerin with a small quantity of suspended sulfur. The mixture is applied to the hair daily, and color gradually develops as a result of the conversion of the colorless lead salt to brownish oxides and sulfides.

The advantages of this procedure are that few people become allergic to the products and the change in color occurs over time, making it possible to introduce a more attractive hair color slowly.

The disadvantages include the fact that the silver dyes have a greenish cast, the copper dyes turn red, hair is often dulled by these products (shine is eliminated because the metal precipitates on the hair cuticle), the smell is often offensive, and the chemical deposits on the hair shafts preclude the use of permanent-wave solutions or permanent color.

Natural Colorants

Henna is a natural hair-coloring product. It is prepared from the dried leaves and flowers of the *Lawsonia alba* plant, which contains an orange dye.

Henna is utilized by mixing the powdered plant pack with hot water and applying it to the hair, resulting in an orange-red coloration that is very resistant to shampooing. The basic color created by the henna preparation is generally considered somewhat unnatural and brassy. But the limitation in henna shades is sometimes overcome by the addition of indigo logwood and chamomile flavone.

The natural aspects of henna (it is noncarcinogenic and nonallergenic) make it popular. However, it is important to check the label on any henna product to make sure that no permanent dyes or peroxides have been added.

Semipermanent Colorants

Low-molecular-weight dyestuffs were developed in the 1950s by the cosmetics industry for semipermanent hair color. These products utilize a mixture of red, yellow, blue, and orange dyes in a thickened shampoo base. They combine to produce natural-looking shades. Unlike the dyes in temporary products, the semipermanent compounds penetrate the cortex of the hair shaft. The major purpose of these products is to brighten dull hair or cover gray. They are also used to produce gold or auburn highlights.

Semipermanent dyes are available as lotions or foams, and are relatively easy to apply. (They are usually left in place for 30 minutes, then rinsed out.) It is possible to have allergic reactions to these products (although this happens less frequently than with permanent dyes), so patch testing is necessary before the first use.

Permanent Colorants

Permanent dyes are by far the largest part of the hair-coloring market. In fact, 90 percent of European and

80 percent of American hair-color sales are permanent colorants. These products are the most popular because of the versatility they allow; hair can be darkened or lightened to virtually any shade, and gray can be completely covered.

Bleaching the hair using hydrogen peroxide was first demonstrated at the Paris Exposition in 1867. In 1883 Monnet, a scientist, patented a process for coloring human hair by treating it with a freshly prepared mixture of p-phenylenediamine and hydrogen peroxide. Today this combination remains the basis of permanent hair coloring or oxidative dyeing.

Hydrogen peroxide lightens the natural color of hair (dark pigments are affected more readily than red shades) or removes artificial color molecules created by permanent dyeing (thus preparing the hair for another color or just changing the hair color). It actually works by causing the release of oxygen from the hair shaft; the more oxygen released, the lighter the hair becomes.

Permanent hair coloring works by increasing the porosity of the hair cuticle and allowing penetration of the hair shaft. The molecules of color are small enough to penetrate the cortex of the hair. Once the color base ingredients begin to interact, they form molecular pigment chains that are too large to pass out of the cuticle. This process can be accomplished in either one or two steps.

The one-step process permanently darkens hair. For this process to be successful, the initial use of a conditioner or filler is required, both to even hair cuticle irregularities and to ensure that the dye is taken up evenly.

The two-step process involves lightening or

bleaching the natural hair color with a mixture of hydrogen peroxide and ammonia, then applying the desired shade or tint.

There can be modifications in the second procedure. *Highlighting,* for example, is the application of the two-step process to selected areas of hair over the entire scalp. *Tipping* lightens only the ends of small groups of hair. *Streaking* involves lightening large clumps of hair. *Frosting* is the process of lightening the entire hair shaft of many individual hairs.

Permanent hair-coloring processes, either bleaching or dyeing, usually last for four to six weeks, with touch-ups or redyeing only necessary to cover new proximal hair growth *(roots)*.

Allergic reactions are possible with most permanent hair-coloring products. For this reason, a patch test is necessary before application. Carcinogenicity has also been reported as a complication of permanent dye preparations. And it should be noted that, although at-home permanent hair dyes are very popular, these products cannot alter the natural hair color more than several shades. For a more dramatic change, an individual needs to go to a professional hairstylist. Professional procedures may also be necessary to cover extensive quantities of gray hair.

Color Cellophanes

Recently, in an attempt to avoid the carcinogenicity of permanent dyes, a new type of coloring technique has been developed, color cellophanes. These cellophanes are blends of primary colors made of certified food drugs and cosmetic-grade color. They are semipermanent if left on the hair for 10 to 15 minutes and permanent if left on for 30 minutes under heat. If peroxide is added to these products, they become truly permanent.

Cautions

Although it appears very easy to color hair today, there are potential problems with the use of any product that physically alters the natural balance of the hair shaft.

Hair porosity varies. Some people have very porous hair that takes color immediately. Others may find it more difficult for their hair to accept color because the hair shaft is very tightly knit, a quality that is usually genetic. (This kind of hair is said to have resistant porosity.) Any color change in this kind of hair requires increased heat or time.

The porosity of hair can vary from strand to strand, resulting in greater absorption of the color by one area and only slight absorption by another and creating an imbalance of color.

The quality of the hair can also affect the way it takes color. For example, fine hair, which has a small diameter, will become saturated with color more quickly than thick hair. But coarse hair that is very porous will process faster than fine hair that is not porous. In addition, if the hair cuticle is damaged by mechanical insult, it is difficult, no matter what type of hair you were born with, to predict how your hair will accept coloring. It is, in fact, important that the uniqueness of each person's hair be taken into account before any hair-color procedure is undertaken.

Other factors can also determine how successful hair coloring will be. Heat from too much blow drying can affect the way a hair color appears, as can sunlight, chlorine from swimming pools, and even the physical trauma that results from too much brushing and combing.

It should be noted that bleaching is the most damaging of all hair-color procedures, because the protein-stripping action of the hydrogen peroxide causes the hair to lose 2 to 3 percent of its weight, which results in dull, unmanageable, easily tangled hair that is brittle and weak.

Permanent colorants are the most damaging hair dyes, because, for a new hair color to be produced, there must be oxidation of the molecules in the hair shaft. The increased porosity resulting from the application of a permanent dye makes hair more susceptible to the effects of static electricity and humidity. It also disrupts the smooth hair shaft surface, making it more difficult to untangle the hair. Both these factors contribute to the brittleness of dyed hair, which predisposes it to breakage.

When either bleaching or permanent dyeing is undertaken, hair should receive extra care. These pampering procedures can include the use of gentle shampoos, light brushing, avoidance of sunlight, additional use of conditioners, and a waiting period before any other chemical procedure, such as permanent waving or straightening, is carried out.

COSMETIC CAMOUFLAGE

The perception of thick hair is based on the distance hair stands from the scalp and from other hairs. That is, the look of fullness can be created by curling the hair using a permanent, which lifts the hair and bends it over, thus covering more exposed skin area. With a round brush and a blow dryer, the hair can be lifted and turned slightly, giving the impression of fullness. Women can also tease (back-comb) their hair to add fullness and the appearance of body. However, if teasing is overdone, it can defeat its purpose by disrupting the hair cuticle and accelerating hair breakage.

Styling aids can also give lift and fullness, simply because their application adds body to the hair shaft and makes it possible for it to stand up rather than lie flat.

Coloring agents are also effective in camouflaging alopecia. If the thinning hair is noticeably darker than the scalp beneath it, hair loss will be more apparent. Lightening the hair makes for less contrast between the scalp and hair, so that the hair loss is less noticeable. It is also possible to dye the scalp with vegetable colorings that match the hair, tattoo the hair pigment onto the scalp, or color the balding area using a pigmented wax pencil.

14

Hair-Care Devices

There are almost as many types of combs, brushes, hair dryers, and other appliances as there are types of hair-grooming aids. Basically, however, the most important devices for keeping hair in shape are combs, brushes, hair dryers, and curling irons.

∽
COMBS

The primary purpose of a comb is to arrange and train the hair into a particular style. Combs are also helpful in cleansing the hair; regular combing will remove dirt and debris from the scalp as well as the hair. Sadly, the best kind of comb, because of its give and substance, is made of tortoiseshell. However, because many tortoises are endangered species, combs made from their shells are not recommended, any more than are those of ivory or horn, both of which also make excellent combs. Instead, good substitutes made from other materials can be found.

Today most commercially produced combs are plastic, hard rubber, or metal.

Plastic Combs

Plastic combs are created by placing the plastic in a mold that hardens. The care with which this procedure is done makes a difference in the final product. For example, in poorly made plastic combs, mold lines are left in the center of each tooth, which results in sharp edges that can cut the hair shaft, scratch the head, and actually remove cellular fragments from the scalp. Poorly made plastic combs also can turn soft when left wet. Better-made plastic combs are safer for the scalp and more resilient.

Hard Rubber Combs

Hard rubber combs are actually made from a hard rubberlike plastic called vulcanite. These combs can be very flexible, durable, and efficient.

Metal Combs

Metal combs are perhaps the least beneficial. They may be durable, but the rigidity of metal makes them hard on the scalp and hair.

A good comb should have even, somewhat dull teeth. The best kind for most people has a saw cut arrangement of teeth, in which the teeth are cut into the handle and their sharp edges eliminated. A good comb should also have a certain amount of give, so that, as it passes through the hair, it doesn't pull the hair or scrape the scalp.

When the hair is wet, a wide-toothed comb is the best, because it is the least likely to tug or rip tangled hair. When the hair is dry, a fine-toothed comb is acceptable.

Combs should be cleaned regularly, particularly if the user suffers from any kind of scalp disorder. Dirt or scalp cells left on the comb's teeth will be placed back on the scalp during the next combing.

BRUSHES

At one time brushing was the primary method by which most people cleansed their hair and scalp. However, because shampooing is more fashionable now, brushes are used to cleanse the hair only between shampoos, and, like combs, to arrange or style the hair.

Brushes have either natural or synthetic bristles. Each has its advantages.

Natural Bristle Brushes

Natural bristle brushes, usually made of animal hair, are excellent for cleansing and polishing the hair, because the bristles are coarse and set unevenly into the handle, which results in a deeper and more thorough brushing.

Synthetic Bristle Brushes

Synthetic bristle brushes (usually nylon or plastic) are best when the hair is wet, particularly if a blow dryer is being used. The bristles on these brushes slip through the hair more easily and don't pull or damage tangled hair or combine with the heat of the blow dryer to stretch the hair.

Brushing can be helpful in lifting the hair to make it appear fuller and to camouflage balding areas. And brushing regularly does stimulate the scalp and give the hair shine and highlights.

However, excess brushing can be damaging. There are cases of hair loss resulting from too vigorous and constant brushing. And anyone who has an excessively oily scalp may find that repeated and prolonged brushing will exacerbate this condition.

HAIR DRYERS

Hair dryers have come a long way since the old days, when large, cumbersome cases attached to electrocutionlike cords were placed on people's heads at the beauty parlor.

Currently there are three kinds of hair dryers: salon hood, home hood, and hand held.

Salon Hood

This is the modern version of the old-fashioned dryer. Made of metal and plastic, salon hoods usually offer a wide range of heat settings.

Although many professional hairstylists now use hand-held dryers, many salons still employ the salon hood, particularly when doing permanents. If a salon does use the hood, it is important to realize that the stylist may leave a patron under the dryer much longer than necessary simply because he or she is not yet ready to proceed. It is, however, detrimental to the hair to allow it to be overdried. The client should request removal of the heat source as soon as the hair feels dry.

Home Hood

This is a simplified version of the salon hood, and, although the heat in a home hood rarely becomes as great as that provided by a salon hood, it is equally important that the home hood be removed when the hair is dry.

Hand Held

For both professional and home use, the hand-held dryer is the most popular on the market. Hand-held dryers have been in existence for only 20 years; however, the range of products, prices, and styles is enormous.

Basically, although it is possible to buy hand-held dryers that offer very high levels of heat, it is best to use 1,000 watts or less to protect the hair and scalp.

If a person has thick hair and feels that it is necessary to use the highest setting to dry the hair, the temperature should be reduced once the hair has dried. It is not necessary to keep the dryer on high for styling, and doing so can be harmful to the hair. It is healthier to allow hair to dry to a damp state naturally; then you can style the hair with the dryer's heat regulator on a very low setting.

For the most part, the attachments, brushes, nozzles, and so on that come with hand-held hair dryers are not of the best quality and are rarely of use.

Despite all the advances in professional and personal hair-drying appliances, the best method has always been, and remains, simply allowing the hair to dry naturally.

∽

CURLING DEVICES

Curling devices use heat to set the hair in a determined style. No solutions are used; heat alone realigns the hair molecules. There are two popular options: the curling iron, which is a hand-held wand, and electric heat curlers that are attached to spikes and a temperature-controlled base. For the most part, the curling irons and electric curlers are used for touch-ups, although some individuals style their entire head with these appliances. Regardless of how much of the hair is treated with a curling iron or electric curlers, certain precautions need to be taken to protect the hair and scalp.

1. To avoid breakage and extensive damage to the hair, the heat of the curling iron should never exceed 270°F. A good curling iron has a temperature gauge with an automatic shutoff at that point.
2. The curling iron should have holes for steam, and be coated with a substance, such as Teflon, that protects the hair.
3. The hair should be slightly damp when either a curling iron or electric curlers are used. Often individuals wash their hair and dry it thoroughly before using these devices. However, if the hair is left damp, the set will hold better and there is less chance of damaging the hair shafts.

In general, electric curlers should be applied to the hair for 15 minutes on a strong setting. The heat should then be turned off and the curlers allowed to cool slightly before removal. A good rule is that the first curler put on should be the first one removed.

15

Personal Hair Care

As part of a living organism, hair is susceptible to the same internal and external forces that affect the rest of the body. The condition of a person's hair depends on his or her general health—both physical and mental—diet, and even the amount of sleep regularly gotten. Also, the environment has a great deal of impact on hair; pollutants in the air, seasonal changes, overall climate all affect the condition, shape, and health of hair. Consequently, how a person cares for his or her hair may have to vary from season to season, or even from place to place.

Regardless of how often a person needs to shampoo, condition, cut, or restyle his or her hair, four basic tenets—shampooing, brushing, cutting, and styling—make hair look its best.

SHAMPOOING

The best shampoo begins with the hair as wet as possible. The hotter the water, the more open the hair follicles become. Consequently, if an individual's hair is very dirty and has a buildup of hair spray (which coats the hair and is resistant to shampooing), then the water should be as hot as possible. If the hair is only moderately dirty, warm or tepid water is better and healthier for the scalp.

Once the hair is thoroughly drenched, a shampoo chosen for the hair type and condition (medicated, conditioning, gentle, protein, and so on) should be applied.

The hair should be massaged in a circular motion. This activates the oil glands and loosens dead scales on the scalp. The hairlines and ends of the hair should receive particular attention.

The hair should be rinsed thoroughly to remove all traces of shampoo. In fact, even after it appears that the shampoo is completely gone, it is not a bad idea to rinse the hair again. Follow the regular rinse with a cold rinse to impart shine to the hair and mediate the trauma of the hot water and massage.

A conditioner can be used at this point.

Next, squeeze the water out of the hair with a towel (do not rub vigorously). Comb to remove tangles, and leave the hair for a few moments before using other drying tools or methods.

∽
BRUSHING

Provided the hair is healthy and brushing is not overdone, this procedure can both help clean and add shine and volume to hair.

When brushing the hair, the bristles should be

pressed on the hair, close to, but not actually touching, the scalp.

Divide the hair into sections, and brush it forward, passing the brush firmly through the full length of the hair and moving the wrist in a semicircular motion with each stroke.

∽
CUTTING

A haircut is, of course, designed to maintain a neat, well-groomed appearance. It can also be directed toward achieving a particular style, flattering positive features of the face and head, minimizing negative aspects (for example, individuals with large noses can wear their hair longer and fuller; conversely, people with small noses might choose to wear their hair shorter), or helping to hide or cover baldness.

The best cut for each individual depends on the texture of the hair and the direction in which it grows. It is important to keep in mind the basic condition of the hair when getting a haircut. To complete a regular haircut, most professional hairstylists use scissors between 4 and 7½ inches in length (smaller scissors are for exact cutting, larger for removing longer hair). And for most people this is the best tool. It is particularly important that people who have thin, damaged, or sparse hair avoid any unusual or peculiar technique, such as razor cuts or slithering-scissor cuts (sliding open scissors up and down hair), which can remove volume and body.

For a person suffering from baldness, the basic

blunt cut, in which the hair is sectioned into five areas and then trimmed straight across, is often helpful in giving the appearance of volume and fullness.

ဆ
STYLING

The old-fashioned method by which many men style their hair to cover baldness is to grow the side hair long, then comb it over the top. This rarely fools anyone, however.

In reality, no hairstyle using only the remaining hairs on an individual's head can completely and naturally camouflage hair loss. However, making the best use of remaining hair is usually accomplished by curling and lifting the hair.

Women may employ other methods, such as finger waving. This is a technique in which damp hair is curled and set around an individual's finger. Finger waving causes the hair to bend into itself and look fuller. However, if the finger waves are too tight, the style may actually point up the sparsity of the hair.

Pin curling usually creates flat curls by twisting damp hair and holding it in place with bobby pins. The resultant curls can overlap or be styled to stand up which helps give the appearance of fullness. However, this style, like finger waves, runs the risk of tightness.

There is no reason not to try to camouflage or cover hair loss. But it is vital to realize the limitations of cosmetic cover-ups.

16

Future Trends and Unapproved Treatments

∽
TEST-TUBE HAIR

New advances in hair-growth research continue to evolve. A better understanding of the basic causes of hair loss should lead to more effective treatment. Recently, scientists at Cambridge University have grown hair in a test tube. Working with samples of skin left from plastic surgery operations, they have developed procedures for extracting hair follicles without damaging the roots. This was done by carefully slicing away the top two layers of skin to bare the hair follicles, which were extracted with fine tweezers and grown in a synthetic blood substitute.

According to the research information, the hair grows at the same rate of 0.037 inches a day as human hair and in the same shape.

This development is not, in itself, a signal that a

cure for baldness is around the corner. However, it provides a medium for new experiments and could lead to an effective treatment for baldness within 10 years. It is now possible to test chemicals on hair without worrying about the toxicity problems associated with testing on humans.

∽
SCALP SHOCKING

According to Stuart Maddin of the University of British Columbia, scalp shocking, a pulsed electronic stimulation, has been shown to grow hair. In this procedure, a hood fits over the head and emits a safe electrical field. Thirty of 56 patients receiving electrical stimulation sprouted new hair, and 66 percent of the test group showed an increased number of hairs.

Scalp shocking is not, however, an accepted or recommended treatment at this time.

∽
IAMIN—GREEK "HEALING CURE"

Loren Pickart, a researcher at the University of California, discovered that a compound previously used to heal wounds might be of value in alleviating baldness. The treatment derives from a chain of three amino acids found in blood, urine, and saliva that binds with copper and triggers the body's natural healing mechanism. In 1986, Pickart found that IAMIN grew clumps of hair on test mice. In 1991, at the University of Wisconsin, Hideo Uno demonstrated that the application of this "healing-cure" compound was 20 times more effective than minoxidil in growing hair.

IAMIN is not on the market at this time.

⌒

HYALURON

This compound provides the substances that the hair follicle normally needs to sustain the growth of healthy hair. Included in Hyaluron are several active components, each of which is believed to influence various biological and cellular factors that contribute to the growth or loss of hair. The three major active components are hyaluronic acid, clycoprotein, and amino acids. Hyaluron also contains thioglycan, a mixture of natural mucopolysaccharides (sugars such as chondroitin sulfate and heparin sulfate) and tetrohydrofurfurylnicotinate, a cutaneous vasodilator (dilates blood vessels), as well as sodium pantothenate and biotin, a member of the B vitamin group, along with topical vehicle additives, such as propylene glycol, sorbic acid, ethanol, distilled water, and perfuming agents. Hyaluron functions as an anti-inflammatory agent; in other words, it claims to reduce the accumulation of skin lipids, which adversely affect hair growth, and increases skin elasticity and cutaneous circulation and respiration.

In a European study, the new preparation was felt to be able to slow the rate of hair loss usually observed in men with male pattern baldness; however, its role in growing hair was considered uncertain.

An American study found that the number of scalp hairs in the nongrowing hairs decreased by 16 percent in the treated group at the end of six months, compared with a 6 percent decline in the placebo group. The number of hairs lost during a standardized daily combing test decreased by 59 percent in the men who applied the new preparation, compared with a 16 percent loss in the placebo group. This study also showed that the extent of hair loss continued to decline significantly between 60 and 90 days in the treatment group, as opposed to no improvement in the placebo group.

Hyaluron is not on the market at this time.

SERATIA MARCESCENS EXTRACT

A new cancer drug, Seratia marcescens extract, has recently been reported to have some effect on chemotherapy-induced hair loss. This breakthrough was presented by Arthur P. Bertolino at the New York University Advances in Dermatology meeting. It appears that Seratia marcescens extract, currently being used in phase II clinical trials for the treatment of recurrent primary brain tumors and prostate cancer, successfully prevents hair loss when used in conjunction with other drugs. The exact way the drug works is still unknown, but there appears to be a noticeable difference in the health of the hair follicle when the extract is used to combat cancer.

Not all work on hair loss is on androgenetic alopecia. All forms of hair loss and baldness are continually being investigated for a number of reasons, including the simple cosmetic aspects of the condition, the possible links between hair disorders and other underlying systemic conditions, and the potential that the discovery of a cure for baldness will open the way to the treatment of other androgen-dependent diseases. In addition, new means to cover balding areas caused by either androgenetic alopecia or alopecia brought about by other conditions are constantly being discovered.

Until a cure for alopecia has been uncovered, there are new and interesting methods by which a person can camouflage hair loss.

As we approach the twenty-first century, the challenge of dealing with hair loss continues. Progress is being made as increasing numbers of scientists are beginning to understand the hair growth and loss system in detail. New tools of biochemistry and molecular biology are identifying key cells, proteins, and genes that control the growth, death, and regeneration of hair. All these factors are helping us better understand many of the underlying conditions that precipitate hair loss, the causes of hereditary androgen-dependent hair loss, and the underlying changes in hair growth that occur throughout adulthood. A hair and its follicle make up one of the most complex systems in the body. How close are we to finding the cure for baldness? Certainly closer than we were a decade ago. Utilizing hair transplant techniques, coupled with exciting new hair-growth-promoting agents, doctors can now hope to restore and ultimately maintain hair growth.

GLOSSARY

Alkalinity   Having a basic pH.

Alopecia   Hair loss from any cause.

Alopecia areata   Hair loss characterized by discrete patches with possible autoimmune cause.

Alopecia totalis   Form of alopecia areata in which hair loss is over the entire scalp.

Alopecia universalis   Form of alopecia areata in which hair loss is over the entire body.

Anagen   Growing phase of the hair cycle.

Anagen effluvium   Hair loss characterized by shedding of actively growing or anagen hairs. Can be caused by chemotherapy agents.

Androgen   Male hormone that, among other functions, regulates growth of the hair follicle.

Androgenetic alopecia   Hereditary loss of hair, which is felt to be at least partially caused by androgen influences.

Anterior scalp   Frontal part of the head.

Axillary hair   Underarm hair.

Bacteria   Microorganisms capable of causing disease.

Biopsy   Testing of a sample piece of tissue.

Chemotherapy   Treatment with drugs that interfere with the division and metabolism of cells.

Cicatricial alopecia   Hair loss asociated with scarring changes in the skin of the scalp.

Congenital   From birth.

Cortex   Outer coating of the hair shaft.

Cuticle   Outer nonliving coating of the hair, made of protein, which gives the hair shine and contributes to its strength.

Dandruff   Scaling on the scalp.

Dermatitis   Inflammation characterized by redness, scaling, and oozing.

Dermatologist   A physician who specializes in skin diseases.

Dihydrotestosterone (DHT)   Metabolite of testosterone felt to play a major role in genetic hair loss.

Dinitrochlorobenzene (DNCB)   Sensitizing chemical used to treat alopecia areata.

Donor site   Area at the back of the scalp from which hair used for transplants is harvested.

Double-blind study   Scientific study in which neither the investigator nor the subjects know who is getting the test material and who a placebo.

Edema   Fluid swelling in the tissues.

Endocrine system   System of hormone-producing glands.

Enzyme Proteins that accelerate specific chemical reactions at body temperature.

Estrogen Hormone that stimulates the development of female secondary sexual characteristics.

5 alpha reductase Enzyme that converts testosterone to its active metabolite.

Flap Piece of tissue partly severed from its place of origin and moved to another location as part of surgical reconstruction.

Follicle Anatomical cavity.

Friction alopecia Hair loss associated with chronic rubbing.

Genetic baldness Hereditary hair loss.

Hair bulb Protrusion of the lowest part of the hair follicle structure, in which the matrix—the actively reproducing component of the hair—is enclosed.

Hair shaft Central hair structure.

Hair transplant Transfer of grafts of hair-bearing tissue from a donor site to recipient balding areas, which subsequently grow hair.

Hirsutism Presence of excessive body and facial hair in physiological locations, especially in women; may be present in normal adults as an expression of an ethnic characteristic or may develop in children or adults as the result of a metabolic disorder, usually endocrine in nature.

Hormone Product of living cells that circulates in body fluids and produces a specific effect on the activity of cells remote from its point of origin.

Hypertension Elevated blood pressure.

Implant   Something inserted into tissue.

Keratin   End product of differentiation of the outer layer of the skin.

Lanugo hair   Dense, cottony or downy growth of early immature hairs.

Lateral scalp   Outer aspects of the scalp.

Lupus   Autoimmune (collagen vascular) disease associated with hair loss.

Male pattern baldness   Common familial baldness.

Matrix   Active growing part of the hair follicle.

Medulla   Inner lining of the hair follicle.

Melanin   Pigment (color) produced in the skin by active cells called melanocytes.

Metabolic   Relating to the physical and chemical processes by which an organism sustains itself.

Microplugs   One to two hair-bearing grafts used in a hair transplant.

Miniplugs   Three to four hair-bearing grafts used in a hair transplant.

Minoxidil   High blood pressure drug utilized as a topical hair-promoting agent.

Ophiasis   A form of alopecia areata in which the loss of hair occurs in bands partially or completely encircling the head.

Papilla   Lower part of the hair follicle, which encases the matrix.

Patch test   Method of testing the allergen nature of substances by placing them on the skin.

pH   Measure of acidity or alkalinity.

Pigment   Substance that imparts color.

Plug   Graft of tissue utilized in hair transplants.

Posterior scalp   Back of the head.

Progesterone   Hormone involved in the female system of sexual reproduction.

Protein Naturally occurring complex of amino acids.

Pubic hair Hair covering the pelvic genitalia.

PUVA Ultraviolet light treatment incorporating psoralen, a substance that binds DNA and long-wave ultraviolet light.

Recipient site Area to which hair transplant grafts are moved.

Root Area of fixation of the hair.

Scalp Part of the head of both sexes containing hair-bearing skin.

Scalp reduction Surgical procedure that removes areas of balding scalp.

Scalp stretching Extension, utilizing scalp expanders, of areas of balding scalp to be removed.

Sebaceous gland Sebum-producing gland attached to the hair follicle.

Seborrhea Flaking on the scalp.

Seborrheic dermatitis Scaling, redness, and inflammation of sebaceous glandular areas.

Senescent alopecia Loss of hair associated with the normal aging process.

Spironolactone Antiandrogen with possible therapeutic potential in genetic hair loss.

Steroid Compound including various hormones involved in the regulation of cell metabolism.

Systemic Pertaining to or affecting a particular group of organs of the body.

Tinea capitis Fungal infection of the scalp.

Telogen Resting phase of the hair cycle.

Telogen effluvium Hair loss secondary to an insult that recycles hair into a resting phase.

Terminal hair Hair in the mature end stage; pigmented hair.

Testosterone Hormone produced by the testes that regulates male sexual characteristics.

Thyroid Hormone-producing gland that regulates metabolism.

Topical Referring to surface application.

Traction alopecia Hair loss secondary to mechanical damage (chronic pulling).

Trichotillomania Hair loss secondary to self-induced plucking.

Tunnel graft Application of a hair transplant plug at an appropriate angle.

Vellus hair Downy, fine, almost invisible hair.

Vertex Top of the head.

Weaving Formation by interlacing strands.

SELECTED
BIBLIOGRAPHY

<u>PART ONE: HAIR LOSS</u>

1 *How Hair Grows*

Asquitin, R. A. *Chemistry of Natural Protein Fibers.*
London: Wiley, 1977.

Atkinson, S. C., Gormia, F. E., and Imrai, S. A. "The
Diameter and Growth Phase of Hair in
Relation to Age." *British Journal of
Dermatology* 71 (1959): 309.

Barth, J. H. "Normal Hair Growth in Children."
Pediatric Dermatology 4 (1987): 173–84.

Caserio, R. "Microscopic Examinations of Hair
Bulb Types and Casts." *Diagnostic Techniques
for Hair Disorders, Part II* 40 (1987): 321–25.

Cunliffe, W. J., Hall, R., Newell, D. J., and
Stevenson, C. J. "Vitiligo, Thyroid Disease, and
Autoimmunity." *British Journal of Dermatology*
80 (1968): 135.

Duggins, O. H., and Trotter, M. "Changes in

Morphology of Hair During Childhood."
Annals of the New York Academy of Sciences
53 (1951): 569.

DEKES, L. K. "Anthropologische Aspekte der Haar
Farbe." *Huntartz* 31 (1980): 76–81.

GIACOMETTI, L. "The Anatomy of the Human Scalp."
Advances in Biology of Skin 6 (1965): 97.

———. "The Anatomy of the Human Scalp." In
Advances in Biology of the Skin, ed. W.
Montagna, vol. 6, *Aging,* 97–120. Oxford:
Pergamon Press, 1964.

HAMILTON, J. B. "Patterned Loss of Hair in Man:
Types and Incidences." *New York Academy of
Sciences* 53 (1951): 708–28.

IOANNIDES, G. "Alopecia: A Pathologist's View."
International Journal of Dermatology 6 (1982):
316–27.

KEOGH, E. V., and WALSH, R. J. *Rate of Greying of
Human Hair Nature.* London: Blackwell, 1965.

MARSHALL, W. A., and TANNER, J. M. "Variations in
Pattern of Pubertal Changes in Boys." *Archives
of Disease in Childhood* 43 (1970): 13–23.

NATOW, A. "Hair Condition and Hair Body." *Cutis*
43 (1985): 380–83.

NEYZI, O., ALP, H., YAKINDAS, A., and YAKACIKLIS,
C. A. "A Sexual Maturation in Turkish Boys."
Annals of Human Biology 2 (1975): 251–59.

PECARO, V., ASTORE, I., BARMAN, J. M., and ARUJO, C. I.
"The Normal Trichogram in the Child Before
Puberty." *Journal of Investigative Dermatology*
42 (1964): 427–30.

PINKUS, F. "Die normale Anatomie der Haut." In
*Handbuch der Haut und Geschlecht
Skiankheiten,* ed. J. Jodassohn, vol. 1,

Anatomie der Haut, 116–255. Berlin: Verlag van Julius Springer, 1927.

ROBBINS, C. R. *Chemical and Physical Behavior of Human Hair*. New York: Van Nostrand Reinhold, 1979.

ROOK, A. "Hair Colour in Clinical Diagnosis." *International Journal of Medical Science* 2 (1969): 415–27.

SAWAYA, M. R., and HONIA, L. S. "Increased Androgen Binding Capacity in Sebaceous Glands in Scalp of Male Pattern Baldness." *Journal of Investigative Dermatology* 92 (1988): 91–95.

STEGGARDA, M. "Changes in Colour with Age." *Journal of Heredity* 32 (1941): 402–3.

——, and SEIBERT, H. C. "Size and Shape of Head Hair from Six Racial Groups." *Journal of Heredity* 32 (1941): 315–18.

SWIFT, J. A. In *The Histology of Keratin Fibers in Chemistry of Natural Protein Fibers*, ed. R. A. Asquitin. London: Wiley, 1958.

TROTTER, M., and DAWSON, H. L. "The Hair of French Canadians." *American Journal of Physiology and Anthropology* 18 (1934): 443–56.

VAN SCOTT, E. J., E KEL, T. M., and AUERBACH, R. "Determinants of Rate and Kinetics of Cell Division in Scalp Hair." *Journal of Investigative Dermatology* 41 (1963): 269.

WASSERMAN, H. P. *Ethnic Pigmentation*. Amsterdam: Excerpta Medica, 1984.

2 *Common Causes of Hair Loss*

BERGFELD, W. "Etiology and Diagnosis of Androgenetic Alopecia." In *Clinics in*

Dermatology, ed. R. DeVillez, 102–07. Philadelphia: J. B. Lippincott, 1988.

DAWBER, R. "Common Baldness in Women." *International Journal of Dermatology* 20 (1981): 647–50.

HELLER, J. J. "Alopecia Areata: Evaluation and Newer Treatment Modalities." *Journal of Military Dermatology* 21 (1990): 18–26.

KUSTER, W., and HAPPLE, R. "The Inheritance of Common Baldness." *Journal of American Academy of Dermatology* 11 (1984): 921–26.

LUDWIG, E. "Classification of the Types of Androgenetic Alopecia (Common Baldness Occurring in the Female Sex)." *British Journal of Dermatology* 97 (1977): 247–54.

MITCHELL, A. J., and KRUH, E. A. "Alopecia Areata: Pathogenesis and Treatment." *Journal of American Academy of Dermatology* 11 (1984): 763–75.

NELSON, D. A., and SPIELVOGEL, R. L. "Alopecia Areata." *International Journal of Dermatology* 24 (1985): 26–34.

NORWOOD, O. T. "Male Pattern Baldness: Classification and Incidence." *British Medical Journal* 68 (1975): 1365–69.

PRICE, V. H. "Alopecia Areata." *Progress in Dermatology* 25 (1991): 1–7.

SPERLING, L. C. "Transverse Anatomy of Telogen Effluvium." *Journal of Military Dermatology* 2 (1990): 3–9.

3 *Uncommon Causes of Hair Loss*

CAMACHO-MARTINEZ, F., and FERRANDO, J. "Hair Shaft Dysplasias." *International Journal of Dermatology* 27 (1988): 71–79.

DUTTA, A. K., MANDAL, S. B., and SOPLING, W. H. "Surface Temperature of Bald and Hairy Scalp in Reference to Leprosy Affection." *International Journal of Leprosy* (1984): 44–48.

FITZPATRICK, T. B., ELLEN, A. L., WOLFF, K., FRIEDBERG, I. M., and AUSTEN, K. F. *Dermatology in General Medicine*. 3d ed. New York: McGraw-Hill, 1990.

GRAHAM, J. H., JOHNSON, W. C., BURGOUN, C. F., and HELWIG, E. B. "Tinea Capitis." *Archives of Dermatology* 12 (1964): 1204–06.

LUBY, J. P. "Varicella Zoster Virus." *Journal of Investigative Dermatology* 61 (1973): 212.

WHITING, D. A. "Structural Abnormalities of the Hair Shaft." *Journal of American Academy of Dermatology* (1987): 1–25.

ZUCKERMAN, A. "Parasitological Review of Current Status of the Immunology of Blood and Tissue Parasites." *Experimental Parasitology*, 1975.

PART TWO: OTHER HAIR AND SCALP PROBLEMS

4 *Local Diseases of the Hair and Scalp*

DAWBER, R. and Rook, A., eds. *Diseases of the Hair and Scalp*. London: Blackwell, 1990.

FISHER, A. A. "Management of Hairdressers Sensitized to Hair Dyes or Permanent Wave Solutions." *Cutis* 43 (1989): 316.

MCKEE, P. H. *Pathology of the Skin*. 1st ed. London: Gower, 1989.

PARISH, L. C., WITKOWSKI, J. A., and MILLIKAN, L. E. "Pediculosis Capitis and the Stubborn Nit." *International Journal of Dermatology* 28 (1988): 436.

RATZER, E. R., and STRONG, E. W. "Squamous Cell Carcinoma of the Scalp." *American Journal of Surgery* 114 (1967): 510.

WYATT, E., and RIGGOTT, J. M. "The Influence of Psoriasis on Hair Diameter." *British Journal of Dermatology* 115 (1981): 96.

5 *Systemic Conditions Affecting the Scalp*

ABOU-MOURAD, N. N., FOSCH, F. S., and STEEL, D. "Dermatopathic Changes in Hypozincemia." *Archives of Dermatology* 1115 (1979): 956–58.

BAUM, E. W., SAMS, W. M., JR., and PAYNE, R. R. "Giant Cell Arteritis: A Systemic Disease with Rare Cutaneous Manifestations." *Journal of the American Academy of Dermatology* 6 (1982): 1081–88.

GOTTE, D. K., and ODOM, R. B. "Alopecia in Crash Dieters." *JAMA* 235 (1976): 262–63.

LYNFIELD, Y. "Effect of Pregnancy on the Human Hair Cycle." *Journal of Investigative Dermatology* 35 (1960): 323–27.

MOCK, D. M., DELORIMER, A. A., LIEBERMANN, N., and METZ, L. "Biotin Deficiency: An Unusual Complication of Parenteral Nutrition." *New England Journal of Medicine* 304 (1981): 820–23.

PROTTERY, C., HARTOP, P. J., and PRESS, M. "Correction of the Cutaneous Manifestations of Essential Fatty Acid Deficiency in Man by Application of Sunflower Seed Oil to the Skin." *Journal of Investigative Dermatology* 64 (1978): 228–34.

SPENCER, L. V., and CALLEN, J. P. "Hair Loss in Systemic Disease." *Dermatology Clinics* 5 (1987): 560–70.

6 *Unwanted Hair*

CUSAN, L., DUPONT, A., BELANGER, A., TREMBLAY, R., MANTES, G., and LABRIE, F. "Treatment of Hirsutism with the Pure Antiandrogen Flutamide." *Journal of the American Academy of Dermatology* 23 (1990): 462–69.

DAWBER, R. In *Diseases of the Hair and Scalp*, ed. A. Rook, 233–59. Oxford: Blackwell, 1982.

DRAELOS, Z. D. "Hair Removal Techniques." *Cosmetic Dermatology* 15 (1990): 10–12.

FERRIMAN, D., and GALLWEY, J. D. "Clinical Assessments of Body Hair Growth in Women." *Journal of Clinical Endocrinology and Metabolism* 21 (1961): 1440–47.

FINE, R. "Spironolactive Therapy in Hirsute Women." *International Journal of Dermatology* 28 (1989): 23–24.

JEMEL, G. B. E. "Hypertrichosis Lanuginosa Acquisita." *Archives of Dermatology* 122 (1986): 805–08.

KUEDAR, J., GIBSON, M., and KRUSINSKI, P. A. "Evaluation of Hirsutism." *Journal of the American Academy of Dermatology* 12 (1985): 215–25.

McKNIGHT, E. "The Prevalence of Hirsutism in Young Women." *Lancet* 27 (1988): 268–70.

REDMOND, G. P., BERGFELD, W., GUPTA, M., BEDOCS, N. M., SKIBINSKI, C., and GIDWANI, G. "Menstrual Dysfunction in Hirsute Women." *Journal of the American Academy of Dermatology* 22 (1990): 76–78.

———, GIDWANI, G. P., GUPTA, M. K., BEDOCS, N. M., PARKER, R., SKIBINSKI, C., and BERGFELD, W. "Treatment of Androgenetic Disorders with Dexamethasone and Response Relationship for

Suppression of Dihydroepiandrosterone-sulfate." *Journal of the American Academy of Dermatology* 22 (1990): 91–93.

RENTOUL, J. R. "Management of the Hirsute Woman." *International Journal of Dermatology* 5 (1983): 265–73.

RITTMASTER, R. S., and LORIAUX, R. L. "Hirsutism." *Annals of Internal Medicine* 106 (1987): 65–107.

SIEGEL, S. S., FINEGOLD, D. M., LANES, R., and LEE, P. A. "ACTH Stimulation Tests and Plasma Dihydroepiandrosterone-sulfate Levels in Women with Hirsutism." *New England Journal of Medicine* 323 (1990): 849–53.

ULGERSKY, R., MEHLMAN, I., GLASS, A., and SMITH, C. "Treatment of Hirsute Women with Cimetidine." *New England Journal of Medicine* 323 (1990): 1040–41.

WAGNER, R. F. "Physical Methods for the Management of Hirsutism." *Cutis* 45 (1990): 319–26.

PART THREE: TREATMENTS FOR HAIR LOSS

7 *Unproven Treatments for Hair Loss*

GIACOMETTI, L. "Facts, Legends, and Myths About the Scalp Throughout History." *Archives of Dermatology* 95 (1967): 629–31.

KINGSLEY, P. *The Complete Hair Book.* New York: Grosset & Dunlap/Fred Jordan Books, 1979.

KLIGMAN, A., and FREEMAN, B. R. "History of Baldness: From Magic to Medicine." *Clinics in Dermatology* 6 (1988): 83–88.

LEACH, E. R. "Magical Hair." *Journal of the Royal Anthropological Institute of Great Britain and Ireland* 88 (1958): 147–64.

LEMEOVE, M. "Facts, Legends and Myths About the Scalp Throughout History." *Archives of Dermatology* 95 (1967): 629–31.

MOERMAN, D. G., "The Meaning of Baldness and Implications for Treatment." *Clinics in Dermatology* 6 (1988): 89–92.

8   *Seeking Professional Help*

DEVILLEZ, R. L., and DUNN, J. "Female Androgenetic Alopecia." *Archives of Dermatology* 122 (1986): 1011–15.

KASICK, J. M., BERGFELD, W. F., STECK, W. D., et al. "Adrenal Androgenetic Female-Pattern Alopecia Sex Hormones and the Balding Woman." *Cleveland Clinic Quarterly* 50 (1983): 111–12.

KRAMARCZUK-HARDINSKY, M. "General Evaluation of the Patient with Alopecia." *Dermatology Clinics* 5 (1987): 483–89.

PRICE, U. H. "Office Diagnosis of Structural Hair Anomalies." *Cutis* 15 (1975): 231–40.

STENGEL, F. "Indications and Technique of Biopsy for Diseases of the Scalp." *Journal of Dermatologic Surgery and Oncology* 4 (1978): 170–71.

9   *Treatments for Male Pattern Baldness*

ARAM, H. "Treatment of Female Androgenetic Alopecia with Cimetidine." *International Journal of Dermatology* 26 (1987): 128–38.

BERGFELD, W. F., and REDMUND, G. P. "Androgenetic

Alopecia." *Dermatology Clinics* 5 (1987): 491–500.

BRODLAND, D. G., and MULIER, S. A. "Androgenetic Alopecia (Common Baldness)." *Cutis* 47 (1991): 173–76.

BURLIER, B., and CUNLIFFE, W. J. "Oral Spironolactone Therapy for Female Patients with Acne, Hirsutism, or Androgenetic Alopecia." *British Journal of Dermatology* 112 (1985): 124–34.

JONES, D. B., IBRAHAM, I., and EDWARDS, C. R. W. "Hair Growth and Androgen Responses in Hirsute Women Treated with Continuous Cyproterone Acetate and Cyclical Ethinyl Oetradiol." *Acta Endrocrinologica* 116 (1987): 497–507.

LUCKY, A. "The Paradox of Androgens and Balding: Where Are We Now?" *Journal of Investigative Dermatology* 50 (1988): 99–100.

10 *New Biological Modifiers for Hair Growth*

DEVILLEZ, R. L. "Topical Minoxidil Therapy in Hereditary Androgenetic Alopecia." *Archives of Dermatology* 121 (1985): 197–202.

FIEDLER, V. C. "Minoxidil: Clinical and Basic Research in Perspective." *Seminars in Dermatology* (1987): 6101–07.

GILHAR, A., PILAR, T., and ETZONI, A. "Topical Cyclosporine in Male-Pattern Baldness." *Journal of the American Academy of Dermatology* 23 (1990): 470–72.

KATZ, H. I. "Topical Minoxidil: Review of Efficacy and Safety." *Cutis* 43 (1989): 95–98.

KOPERSKI, J., ORENBERG, E. K., and WILKINSON, D. "Topical Minoxidil Therapy for Androgenetic

Alopecia." *Archives of Dermatology* 123 (1987): 1438–87.

OLSEN, E. S., and DeLONG, E. "Transdermal Viprostol in the Treatment of Male-Pattern Baldness." *Journal of the American Academy of Dermatology* 23 (1990): 470–72.

——, WEINER, M., and AMARA, I. A. "Five-Year Follow-up of Men with Androgenetic Alopecia Treated with Topical Minoxidil." *Journal of the American Academy of Dermatology* 22 (1990): 643–46.

——, WEINER, M. S., DeLONG, E. R., et al. "Topical Minoxidil in Early Male-Pattern Baldness." *Journal of the American Academy of Dermatology* 13 (1985): 185–92.

ROENIGK, H. H. "New Topical Agents for Hair Growth." *Clinics in Dermatology* 6 (1988): 119–27.

——, PEPPER, E., and KUROVILLU, S. "Topical Minoxidil Therapy for Hereditary Male-Pattern Alopecia." *Cutis* 39 (1987): 337–42.

TEREZAKIS, N., and BAZZANO, G. S. "Retinoids: Compounds Important to Hair Regrowth." *Clinics in Dermatology* 6 (1988): 129–31.

VANDERVEEN, E., ELLIS, C., KANG, S., et al. "Topical Minoxidil for Hair Regrowth." *Journal of the American Academy of Dermatology* 6 (1984): 1421.

WEISS, V. C., and WEST, D. D. "Topical Minoxidil Therapy and Hair Regrowth." *Archives of Dermatology* 12 (1985): 191–92.

11 *Surgical Procedures*

ALT, T. H. "Evaluation of Donor Harvesting Techniques in Hair Transplantation." *Journal of Dermatologic Surgery and Oncology* 10 (1984): 799–806.

————. "Hair Transplantation and Scalp Reductions." In *Cosmetic Surgery of the Skin,* 103–46. Philadelphia: B. C. Decker, 1991.

HITZIG, G. S., and SADICK, N. S. "A New Technique of Curvilinear Scalp Reduction." *Journal of Dermatologic Surgery and Oncology* 15 (1990): 1108–17.

KNOWLES, W. R. "Hair Transplantation: A Review." *Dermatology Clinics* 5 (1987): 515–30.

LUCAS, M. "The Use of Minigrafts in Hair Transplantation Surgery." *Journal of Dermatologic Surgery and Oncology* 14 (1988): 1389–92.

MANDERS, E. K., and GRAHAM, W. P., III. "Alopecia Reduction by Scalp Expansion." *Journal of Dermatologic Surgery and Oncology* 10 (1984): 967–69.

NORWOOD, O. T. "Micrografts and Minigrafts for Refining Grafted Hairlines." *Dermatology Clinics* 5 (1987): 545–52.

————. "Predicting Hair Growth for Hair Transplantations." *Journal of Dermatologic Surgery and Oncology* 7 (1981): 477–80.

————. "Scalp Reduction in the Treatment of Androgenetic Alopecia." *Dermatology Clinics* 5 (1987): 531–44.

PINSKI, J. B. "Hair Transplantation." *Seminars in Dermatology* 6 (1987): 249–63.

SADICK, N. S., and HITZIG, G. S. "Adjuvant Techniques in Hair Transplantation." *Journal of Dermatologic Surgery and Oncology* 15 (1990): 1108–17.

STEGMAN, S. J., TROMOVITCH, T. A., and GLOGAU, R. G. "Surgical Management of Alopecia." In *Cosmetic Dermatology Surgery*, 83–143. Philadelphia: Year Book Medical Publishers, 1990.

STOUGH, D. B., and NELSON, B. R. "Incisional Slit Grafting." *Journal of Dermatologic Surgery and Oncology* 14 (1991): 53–60.

UNGER, M. G. "The Modified Major Scalp Reduction." *Journal of Dermatologic Surgery and Oncology* 14 (1988): 80–84.

12 Hair Prosthetics

COLLETTI, A. B. *Competency in Cosmetology.* New York: Keystone, 1987.

COONEY, S., and HARPER, C. *Wigs: A Complete Guide for the Profession.* Englewood Cliffs, N.J.: Prentice-Hall, 1973.

Forbes Magazine (July 22, 1991): 83–87.

KINGSLEY, P. *The Complete Hair Book.* New York: Grosset & Dunlap/Fred Jordan Books, 1979.

MAYHEW, J. "Hair Techniques and Alternatives to Baldness." *Conch Magazine* (1983).

PART FOUR: HAIR CARE

---

13 Hair Cosmetics

BOYLLIN, C. "Shampoos and Hair Conditioners." *Clinics in Dermatology* 6 (1988): 83.

COLLETTI, A. B. *Competency in Cosmetology.* New York: Keystone, 1987.

CORBETT, J. F. "Changing the Color of Hair." In *Principles of Cosmetics for the Dermatologist,*

eds. P. Frost and S. Hurwitz. St. Louis:
C. V. Mosby, 1982.

DRAELOS, Z. K. "Cosmetic Camouflage in Female
Androgenetic Alopecia Patients." *Cosmetic
Dermatology* (1991): 13–15.

————. "Hair Coloring and Curling." *Cosmetic
Dermatology* (September 1990): 6–7.

————. "Hair Cosmetics." *Dermatology Clinics* 9
(1991): 19–27.

FINKELSTEIN, P. "Hair Conditioners." *Cutis* 6 (1970):
542.

GOLDENBERG, R. L. "Hair Conditioners: The
Rationale for Modern Formula." In *Principles
of Cosmetics for the Dermatologist,* eds. P. Frost
and S. Hurwitz, 157–59. St. Louis: C. V. Mosby,
1982.

NATRU, A. J. "Hair Bleach." *Cutis* 17 (1987): 28–30.

O'DONAHOE, M. N. "Hair Cosmetic." *Dermatology
Clinics* 5 (1987): 619–29.

ZAHN, H., and HILTERHAUS, S. "Bleaching and
Permanent Waving Aspects of Hair Research."
Journal of the Society of Cosmetic Chemists 37
(1986): 159

14 *Hair-Care Devices*

COLLETTI, A. B. *Competency in Cosmetology.* New
York: Keystone, 1987.

KENNETH. *Kenneth's Complete Book on Hair.* New
York: Doubleday, 1971.

KINGSLEY, P. *The Complete Hair Book.* New York:
Grosset & Dunlap/Fred Jordan Books, 1979.

ZVIAK, C. *The Science of Hair Care.* New York:
Marcel Dekker, 1986.

Index

DATE DUE